# Jump into Shape

# JUMP INTO SHAPE
## The Fast, Fun Way to Physical Fitness

### SIDNEY FILSON & CLAUDIA JESSUP

*photographs by Bert Torchia*
*illustrations by Jonathan Richards*

*Franklin Watts, Inc.*
*New York | London | 1978*

**to Master Sanford Meisner**
*he taught me to seek the truth of the moment*

**to Master Ron Van Clief**
*he taught me to seek perfection in myself
and my students*

ISBN: 0-531-09902-4

Library of Congress Catalog Card No.: 78–57009
Text copyright © 1978 by Sidney Filson and Claudia Jessup
Photograph copyright © 1978 by Bert Torchia
Illustrations copyright © 1978 by Jonathan Richards
Printed in the United States of America

5 4 3 2 1

# Contents

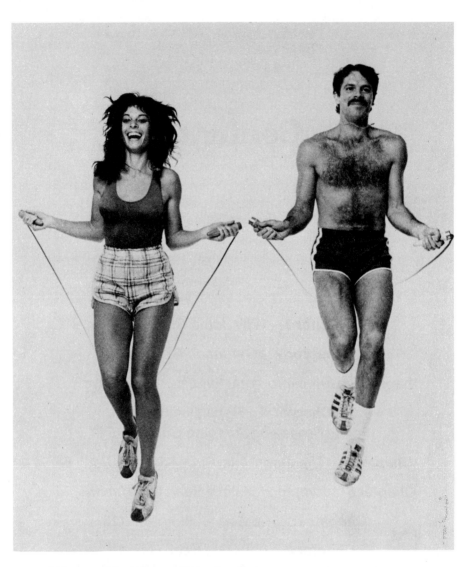

*Sidney and Andy jumped into shape . . .
you will too!*

# Chapter *1*

# *Why Jump Rope?*

*Cinderella, dressed in yellow,*
*Ran upstairs to kiss her fellow.*
*By mistake, she kissed a snake!*
*How many doctors did it take?*
*1,2,3,4,5,6,7,8 ...*
AMERICAN FOLK RHYME, NINETEENTH CENTURY

Jumping rope, for most of us, conjures up visions of kids clustered around jump ropes, whiling away long, lazy summer afternoons. Many of us harbor vague memories of games with names like Double Dutch, Front door/Back door, and Rocking the Cradle. And do you remember Hot Pepper—turning the rope as fast as you can?

Boxers have also popularized rope jumping and use it to build stamina and fancy up their footwork in the ring. They even work out in three-minute segments, with a minute's rest in between, to simulate professional match conditions and develop inner timing.

Jumping rope is also the shortest way possible to a beautiful body. There is *nothing* you can spend less time on and get more results. It's the best way I know to reduce thighs, hips, and buttocks—all those bulges and spreads that are normally the hardest places to trim down.

If you want to be in super shape and bursting with energy, jump rope! I am going to show you exactly how you can jump yourself into shape in just two weeks—*in only fifteen minutes a day*. If you're dieting, you'll lose inches even faster.

Besides shaping your figure and toning your muscles, you will also improve the efficiency of your lungs, blood vessels, and heart. Rope jumping is believed by many physical fitness experts to be better for your heart than jogging. Recent research studies have proven that ten minutes of vigorous rope jumping is equal to thirty minutes of jogging.[1]

"Rope jumping is anything but child's play; it's superb aerobic exercise," says Dr. Richard Stein, director of the coronary heart disease treatment and prevention program at Downstate Medical Center in Brooklyn, New York.

"Aerobic" means that jumping rope not only gets the oxygen flowing through your body, but it also combats circulatory fatigue and promotes overall cardiovascular fitness: the kind of fitness that helps your heart pump more blood with less effort. This overall fitness will keep you healthy and may help you live longer.

Only five minutes of rope jumping per day is the equivalent of a set of tennis (singles) or nine holes of golf. But you should go the full fifteen minutes to give your heart a good workout and to build stamina.

In terms of overall exercise for the cardiovascular system, here is a comparison of rope jumping with other popular forms of exercise and sports:

[1]From a study conducted by John A. Baker: *Comparison of Rope Skipping and Jogging as Methods of Improving Cardiovascular Efficiency of College Men.* (See Bibliography.)

## JUMPING ROPE FOR FIFTEEN MINUTES IS EQUAL TO:*

| | |
|---|---|
| TENNIS | 3 sets (singles) |
| GOLF | 27 holes (without motorized cart) |
| BICYCLING | 3 miles in under 9 minutes |
| SWIMMING | 700 yards in 17 to 23 minutes |
| RUNNING | 1 mile in 8 minutes |
| RUNNING/WALKING | 1½ miles in 15 to 17 minutes |
| SKATING ice/roller | 1 hour |
| SKIING snow/water | 45 minutes |
| VOLLEYBALL | 1 hour |
| FOOTBALL/SOCCER/LACROSSE | 40 minutes (active play) |
| SQUASH/HANDBALL | 30 minutes |
| ROWING | 27 minutes |

*adapted from Kenneth H. Cooper's studies on aerobics

Best of all, jumping rope is fun—and easy, once you get the hang of it and master all of the steps and routines that keep away monotony. You can jump by yourself or with friends, anywhere—indoors or out. In these days when people spend fortunes on athletic club memberships and the latest equipment and snappy sportswear, jumping rope is the ideal exercise for tightening your belt financially as well as physically.

## *JUMPING INTO A NEW FIGURE*

You'll learn later on about the specific therapeutic benefits of jumping rope. Now, let's look at the body benefits from an aesthetic point of view. Pretty or handsome, whatever your goal, it's easy to get there via a jump rope.

> *Let's realign,*
> *Let's redesign,*
> *Jump rope!*

*Let's improve,*
*Let's remove,*
*Jump rope!*

*Let's reshape,*
*Let's remake,*
*Jump rope!*

Beautification of the body is a major benefit of jumping rope. Can you imagine a more enjoyable way to hit so many problem areas at one time?

## A JUMP ROPE IS A GIRL'S BEST FRIEND

Women have their very own trouble spots: hard-to-reach, nasty, lumpy, bumpy areas that build up and refuse to be dieted away. Or, just as disturbing, there are all those spots that simply go slack. The beauty magazines feed spot-reducing and reshaping articles to the feminine market constantly, and with good reason. Now, there's a better way to fight back and beautify your body. Let's get specific:

*Upper Arm.* Hanging flesh on the upper arm is unsightly. It limits clothing choices, and in bathing suit weather there's no way to disguise it. A deposit of cellulite is no better.

Don't despair. Jumping rope *will* shape up your upper arms. Proper form for jumping (see chapter three) requires you to keep your arms quiet, with movement restricted to the wrist only. Don't let that fool you. You'll be working your upper arms like crazy! Jumping rope is controlled, concentrated exercise. You'll love the toning action that results as the newly worked muscle responds, breaks up fatty deposits, and gives a pretty, rounded shape to your arm.

Jumping rope will prevent you from ever developing upper arm problems, if you have been fortunate enough to avoid them thus far.

*Forearms.* Jumping rope will make them tight and nicely curved as they respond to the controlled-wrist action.

*Upper Chest.* This will take on a desirable, rounded firmness as the controlled-wrist action does its quiet job. Rope jumping will build up your pectoral muscles, which will help support your breasts better.

*Shoulders and Upper Back.* These areas will respond to your workouts and you'll never have to worry about "widow's hump" (the rounding of the shoulders that causes a distortion of the upper back). If you are having a posture problem. it will be chased away by your newly toned muscles.

*Buttocks and Thighs.* These bane-of-your-existence areas really get a shake-up when you shape up with a jump rope. These areas are tough to revamp. You need to go into full battle plan to combat unsightly spread. Armed with your rope, you can be confident that the day will arrive when you will look down at your thighs with pride—no more bulging saddle lump. Jump! Your buttocks *will* lift. Keep jumping! The front of your thighs *will* become beautifully chiseled.

*Calves.* Usually underdeveloped on women, they cause the thighs to look even bigger by comparison. Jumping rope will give a balanced beauty to the entire leg. A curvaceous calf is one of the many pluses attributed to the rope.

Fat calves will also be hard hit by the exercise and give way in a short time. Whatever the problem, you can rest assured that your whole leg will be brought into better proportion.

*Stomach and Waist Area.* Your midsection must be dealt with separately. Jumping rope will help bring down your weight, and you may thereby lose some inches off your waist. To reshape your middle, however, specific concentrated exercise is required. (You will learn special stomach exercises in chapter three.)

*Upper Hip.* This area will take on a lanky, lean line. In fact, this is one of the first areas to show the results of rope jumping. So if hips are your particular problem, grab your rope right away!

## MANNING YOUR JUMP ROPE

A jump rope can be a man's best friend, too. Men have their own problem areas, most of which are a result of not working out. Lack of exercise results in underdevelopment, characterized by slack, thin, or flabby areas all over the body. But, lucky males, nature has blessed you with muscles that respond quickly, and you can't find a better exercise than jumping rope.

Specifically, look at these areas:

*Neck (Trapezius).* This area responds well to the controlled-wrist action required for proper form (see chapter three). Your neck will fill out nicely and look sturdy and strong.

*Shoulders and Back (Trapezius).* Jumping rope will straighten you right up and fill these areas out with a strong, muscled look.

*Upper Arm (Deltoid, Biceps, Triceps).* This area gets wonderful action when you jump rope. The development here will be supple and long-lined, never bunchy.

*Forearm (Flexors).* This will develop quickly and show good definition.

*Chest (Pectoralis Major).* This broad, thick, triangular muscle (situated at the upper and fore part of the chest) will spring right into view and round out nicely. Your entire chest area will respond rapidly to jumping rope.

*Hips (Gluteal Region).* These will be quickly affected by jumping rope. The entire area, side and back, will become slim and strengthened.

*Thigh (Pectus in front, Biceps in back).* The entire area will respond immediately and curve right up for strength and good looks.

*Calf (Soleus).* This area has as its superficial layer a powerful muscle mass, which shows terrific response to rope jumping and shapes up beautifully.

So, men, if you're not into pumping iron but want a supple, attractively muscled body, man your jump rope. You'll be delighted with the results.

### EVERYBODY JUMP!

The *Guinness Book of World Records* even salutes rope jumping. The latest endurance record was set in Japan in 1970: Kazuya Shiozaki jumped 49,299 turns in five hours and thirty-seven minutes, without a break or fault!

Don't be discouraged. If you work up to jumping a full fifteen minutes a day, no one will accuse you of being a slacker. You may not break any records, but you'll look great and be fit. Your stamina and coordination will improve, and you'll have more energy.

Jumping rope will help you excel at other sports and exercises, too. Runners and joggers will improve their endurance. (Many runners jump rope on rainy days and during the winter to keep in shape.) Golfers will strengthen their wrists. Squash players will have better hand-eye coordination. Tennis players will move around the court better and change directions quicker. Children, too, will greatly improve their agility at games.

And you're going to have fun while you get into super shape. I'll start you out jumping to music, and before long you'll be dancing on the rope. You'll learn a lot of fancy steps, and I promise that your family and friends will be impressed.

What are you waiting for? Start jumping today, and experience all the good things that are in store for you.

# Chapter 2

# *Getting in Gear*

Jumping rope doesn't require much preparation or equipment. Nevertheless, before you start jumping, here are some words of advice.

### GET YOUR DOCTOR'S OKAY

If you're over thirty-five, have a medical checkup. Jumping rope is fun, but it's strenuous, especially if you have been reasonably inactive. Don't begin any new exercise program without consulting your doctor.

If you have had any lower back problems, arthritis, or have been treated for any orthopedic illness, check with your doctor to make sure jumping rope is healthy for you. Any unusual medical history calls for your doctor's approval before jumping rope.

If you're over forty, or have any doubts about your jumping stamina, don't take any chances: have a stress test. (For more information about stress tests and jumping rope in relation to your heart and general health, see chapter six.) Check with your family physician or local medical center to see who offers stress tests in your area. Lots of "Y"s offer this service, and sometimes schools set up a special program in their gyms. This test is expensive but worth it in the long run. Prices vary from about $100 to $300.

## EQUIPMENT

*The right shoes.* Never jump rope in your bare feet. The rope can catch in your toes and, besides tripping you up, the pain can be stinging. A good shoe is protection for ankle and knee joints. If you're serious about jumping rope, get yourself a pair of lightweight running shoes. There are many good running shoes on the market, but look for ones with a lot of padding under the *ball* of the foot. (Joggers need shoes with padded heels, but rope jumpers are going to be on the balls of their feet all the time.)

A tennis sneaker doesn't offer enough padding for the rope jumper! And sneakers are heavier, which will keep the spring out of your step.

Stick with running shoes. Make sure they fit well, not too loose or tight. It's best to buy them at a store that specializes in sporting goods. The sales people are usually knowledgeable and are willing to spend time fitting you properly.

*The right rope.* Be sure to buy a long rope! A nine-and-one-half-foot rope is the standard long rope measurement and does fine for everyone. If the rope is too long, tie a knot or two until the length is suitable for you. This will help your jumping: the heavier the rope, the easier it will be to turn.

When buying a rope, look for:

• handles that offer a firm grip, with ball bearings that will enable the rope to turn easily without catching or twisting;
• a leather or very heavy natural or synthetic fiber rope that will make turning easier.

Watch out for tricky, gimmicky ropes. There are ropes on the market made out of noodles and all sorts of strange things. The fact that a rope is endorsed by a famous athlete does not necessarily mean that it's right for you. Look out for narrow, flimsy handles that fall apart quickly. Avoid weighted handles, unless you are trying to develop your upper arms substantially and want to work with extra weight.

*Making your own rope.* A lot of people like to do this, and it's perfectly acceptable. At a hardware store, purchase #10 sash cord, which is heavy enough. I have seen people make ingenious loops at the ends of plain rope and do just as well as someone with a fancy boxer's special.

## WHAT TO WEAR

The right outfit for jumping is a matter of personal preference. Anything that's comfortable is fine: don't wear anything that will constrict your circulation. Shorts and T-shirts are great in summer; sweat pants and tops will keep you warm in cooler weather. They all come in a rainbow of colors.

Jumpers who find themselves perspiring profusely should wear head *sweatbands* and *wristbands*. Make sure they are made of cotton terrycloth, so they will absorb the moisture.

Wear *high socks* or *knee socks* because it's important to keep your calf muscles warm. Or wear *leg warmers*, like ballet dancers who know how necessary it is to keep the leg muscles hot.

Women should wear *a good support bra*. Many companies are making athletic bras for women nowadays. An alternative for good chest support is a very tight *leotard top*.

Men should wear good *athletic support*.

## WHAT TO DO ABOUT ACHING MUSCLES

After your first day's jumping workout, you will most likely find yourself with some aching muscles, especially calves. The best treatment is an analgesic rub. I've been told by physical therapists that the brand makes no difference. The heat only penetrates the surface—it's the actual rubbing that is therapeutic. With that in mind, you could rub down with cold cream and get the same effect. I personally feel that a heat rub is comforting to an aching muscle.

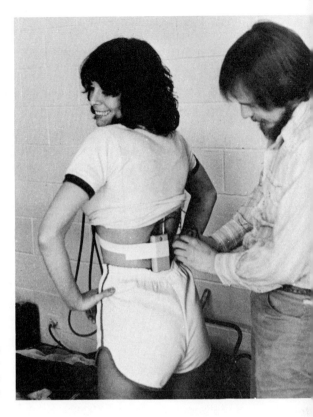

*Filson getting into TV sound gear for ABC's "Contemporary Woman" show*

A *comfrey poultice* can also be most soothing to aching calves. Sore muscles love the beneficial effects of comfrey. Here's how to make it:

- Let steep in a pan of *cold* water: three or four tea bags of comfrey leaf and two tea bags of comfrey root.[1] (If you can find only one or the other, use it anyway.)
- After the comfrey has steeped for about twenty minutes, soak a washcloth in the tea.
- Apply to sore calves. Cover with plastic. Wrap with an ace bandage (not too tight).
- Leave on overnight.

[1]Available at most natural food or herb shops, comfrey is an herb which can be grown fresh in the warm months, or indoors.

## A WORD ABOUT MUSIC

The best way (and as far as I'm concerned, the *only* way) to jump rope is to skip to music. The rhythms and the sounds are going to make your feet fly. Get together some good, fast long-playing records or cassette tapes. Long-playing records are perfect because they'll give you about fifteen minutes to a side, the length of one jumping session. Have a few good 45 r.p.m. records on hand for shorter, faster jumps.

Choose music you enjoy. The beat doesn't always have to be fast-paced, and you'll want to vary it. But keep in mind that mellow love songs and operatic arias just don't make it as jumping tunes.

# Chapter 3

# Jump into Total Fitness ...in 14 Days!

All right, now that you've gotten your gear together, you and your rope are ready for action. My fourteen-day shape-up program will take you only fifteen minutes a day; a mere two weeks to a shapelier, healthier you.

Why not start right now? Assuming you've had a medical checkup and, if you're over forty, a stress test, there's never any better time than the present. Don't procrastinate until the beginning of the week. How often has each of us looked to magical Monday for beginning a new diet or exercise routine? And how many times, unfortunately, has Monday slipped by, all our good intensions fading with it?

But this time it will be different: jumping rope is *fun*. It's also the fastest way I know to total physical fitness. No matter how tight your schedule, you can spare fifteen minutes a day, even if it means getting up that much earlier in the morning. It is your responsibility to take the best possible care of your body and your health. Besides, you reap extra benefits from exercising—you'll feel great, and your surplus energy will radiate into every other area of your life, including your relationships with others.

## WHEN SHOULD YOU JUMP?

I advocate exercising in the mornings, but it's up to you to choose the best time for you. Try to establish a fixed time for jumping, slotted into your regular daily routine. It doesn't matter when you do it, as long as you do it. Remember, however, *do not exercise for an hour and a half after eating*, longer after a heavy meal.

If you're dieting, try to jump for a few minutes before each meal. It won't increase your appetite. On the contrary, you'll feel less hungry. And, of course, you'll be burning up a few extra calories as well.

## WHERE SHOULD YOU JUMP?

Jump anywhere—indoors, outdoors. Once you become proficient, you can jump in a space as small as a closet. You can jump by your desk at the office, in the kitchen while you're waiting for the eggs to boil—any place that's convenient. Try to opt for a wooden surface rather than hard concrete. Jump on a carpeted surface, even if you have to put down a small piece of carpet to jump on. (This is also essential if you want to protect your expensive rugs.)

If you're jumping right (landing lightly on the balls of your feet) and have good shoes to put as much cushioning between you and the surface you're hitting, you have nothing to worry about. No matter what the surface, if you can *hear* your feet hitting the ground you're jumping too hard.

If you jump indoors, keep the windows closed so you can perspire—and you will. Remember, if you don't reach the point where you're perspiring profusely, you're not working hard enough to reap the benefits of the exercise.

## GET READY!

Enough talk, let's get going. Take your phone off the hook, or tell your family you don't want to be disturbed for the next fifteen minutes. Better yet, have them join in—all ages can benefit from jumping rope since it tones, shapes, and improves both coordination and circulation. If you work out together as a family unit, you will spur each other on and keep each other from slacking off or skipping a day. And to top it off, you'll all have fun together.

Before you actually start, you must learn my jumping-rope rules. They'll be repeated often enough, until they become automatic to you. There are just a few, but they are essential:

- Breathe through your *nose only* while jumping.
- Always land on the balls (front) of your feet. Jump as lightly as possible, don't pound.
- Work the rope with your wrists only. Too much arm action will exhaust you and is unnecessary.

In addition, here are a few extra pointers to remember during your daily workout:

- You must always time yourself. As I've said, the easiest way is to put on a long-playing record that gives you approximately fifteen minutes to a side. If music is not available, jump by the clock or kitchen timer.
- When you're not jumping you must stretch. (You'll get specific stretching exercises in the day-by-day program.)
- Don't look down at the rope when you jump; keep your eyes straight ahead.
- Jump only high enough to clear the rope.
- Keep your knees slightly bent—always!
- If you miss the rope or get tangled, try not to stop. While getting the rope back into position, try to keep jumping or dancing in place.
- In the beginning, jump in front of a mirror, if possible. Check out the different reactions each step produces on your body. It's the best way to actually see how jumping rope will tone your muscles.
- When you exercise vigorously, you need supplements of vitamins C and B-complex to replace the water soluble vitamins lost through perspiration. Besides vitamins, be sure to

include raw greens and at least one fresh fruit in your daily diet. (If you want to lose weight, check out my Jump-Into-Super-Shape Diet, chapter five.)

## A WORD TO OLDER JUMPERS

If you're over forty or haven't exercised for a number of years, it's important to start slowly. You will be able to follow this fourteen-day program, because you will have plenty of time for resting (stretching) when you're not jumping. Generally, I let my students jump until they're tired, then stretch themselves until they are ready to jump again. This is similar to "interval training" (see chapter six, page 104), which recommends that you work and rest in sets.

Once you have built your stamina, you will be able to jump for fifteen minutes straight, using the stretching exercises for slow cooling down after the jumping session.

## A WORD TO ALL JUMPERS

It's important to jump every day in the beginning. Later on, after you have built your stamina you can go on a maintenance program of three times a week (alternate days), although it's better for your body to keep in the exercise-every-day habit.

I'll have a lot to say about discipline in this and subsequent chapters, but the accepted maxim is: If you take two days off from exercise there will be a deterioration in your stamina, three days off and you won't go back to the exercise. Don't let this happen!

## A WORD OF WARNING

The easiest way to hurt yourself while jumping rope is to come down too hard on the floor. You must think of your feet as feathers. I've noticed that people are most apt to pound the floor when they are learning a new step. So, test yourself, especially when you are learning new steps. Turn off the music and listen. If you *hear* your feet, you're jumping too hard.

I don't mean to scare you—jumping rope is not a dangerous

exercise. But I find that many of my students damage themselves by not paying enough attention to their own bodies. All it takes is one wrong move for you to damage yourself for a long time; a pulled muscle can last up to six weeks.

So, be in tune with your body. If anything hurts, don't ignore it. See the chart of warning signals and their remedies in chapter six, pages 106–107. When something hurts (and before you blame a previous injury), make sure you're not causing it by pounding.

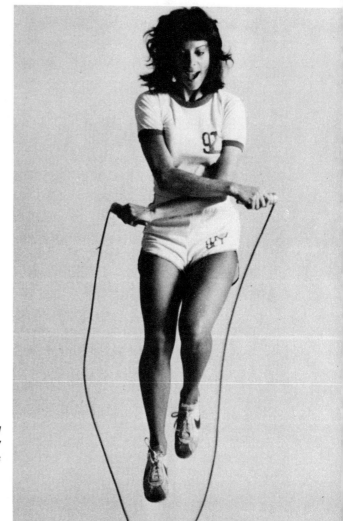

*Start jumping
your way
to total fitness*

## DAY #1

First of all, pick up your rope. Make sure you have a *good grip* on the handles. Don't be tentative. Your *thumbs* should be right on the edge of the handles. Place your *upper arms and elbows* close to your rib cage (touching would be perfect form). Pull your *hands and forearms* back so they are at right angles, straight out from your sides. (This may feel uncomfortable at first, but you'll adjust to it, and it will make your jumping easier.) Keep your *hands* at waist level, not above or below. Your *wrists* should be on the same straight line as your forearms, not tipped back. Make sure your *arms* stay at your sides, not in front of your body. The *rope* should be resting behind your heels on the floor.

When you turn the rope, you want to be the center of a perfect moving circle. You want a continuous turning action. Remember, your wrists turn the rope, not your arms! Rotate your wrists in a circular motion as you turn the rope.

You must be concerned with your form: it will make your jumping easier, and you will look better if you ever attract an audience while jumping rope.

All right. Before you begin to jump, I want to teach you stretching, the way to rest if you get tired.

*Proper Form* ▶

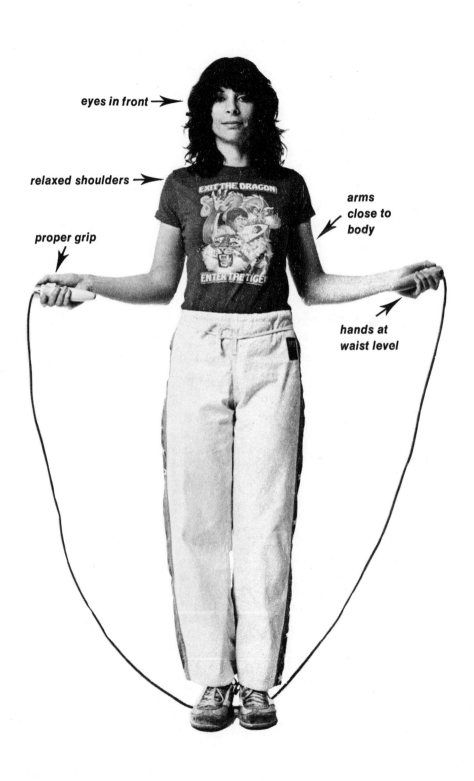

eyes in front →

relaxed shoulders →

arms
close to
body

proper grip

hands at
waist level

### *The Resting Stretch*

Exhale through your mouth, and push *all* the air out of your stomach. Bend over and try to place your palms flat on the floor. Keep your knees straight, locked in place. Just *stay* there. Breathe in through your nose and out through your mouth. Remain relaxed, totally relaxed. You want to stretch the big muscles and your hamstring tendons in the back of your legs.

Once you've reached your deepest stretch, don't retreat from it: stay there. Do not bounce—bouncing is *never* stretching. Keep breathing evenly, in through the nose, out through the mouth.

Whenever you get tired of jumping, the way to rest is to stretch. Do not rest by standing around: you *must* stretch your muscles. Anytime you feel tired, go into this stretch, and stay in this position until you feel collected. Then start jumping again.

During your workout period every day you must be doing *only* two things: *jumping or stretching*.

*The Resting Stretch*

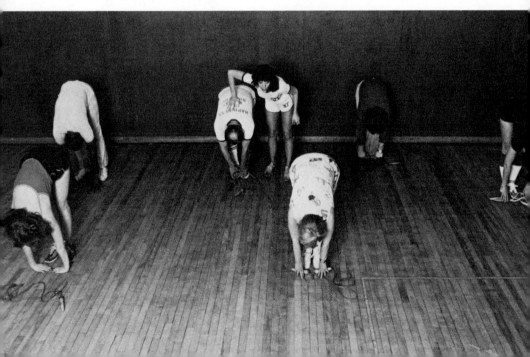

*Learning new steps
is easy when you
hold your rope!*

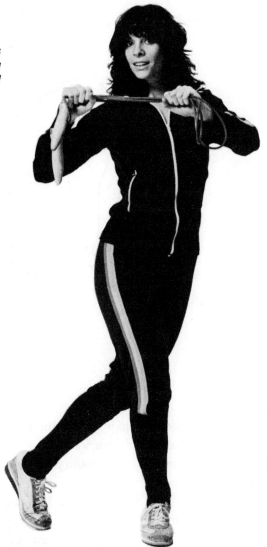

### Practice Position

Take your rope and fold it in half. Hold it in front of your body, chest level. Grip one end with your right hand, the other with your left.

Whenever you are learning a new step, start out in this practice position and work in slow motion. Practice the step without jumping over the rope. Remember, always jump onto the balls of your fee, lightly. If you can *hear* yourself landing, you're jumping too hard.

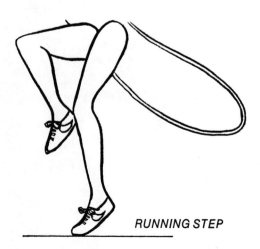

RUNNING STEP

## The Running Step

Jump over the rope lightly onto the ball of your right foot. Jump onto the ball of your left foot.

Now right, now left: running in place over the rope, *with no bounce in between.*

Practice the running step in the practice position, without jumping over the rope. You can go slow; you can go fast. Jump lightly onto the ball of one foot, then the other. Keep your knees high, as if you were a prancing pony.

Now get into the proper jumping position. Make sure you're holding the rope properly—a firm grip on the handles, upper arms close to the body, and forearms and hands straight, at waist level.

Jump: change feet as you run in place over the rope. Remember, there is no bounce in between jumps: jump right, jump left. Don't move forward as you jump, stay in one place. Look in front of you, and think *up.*

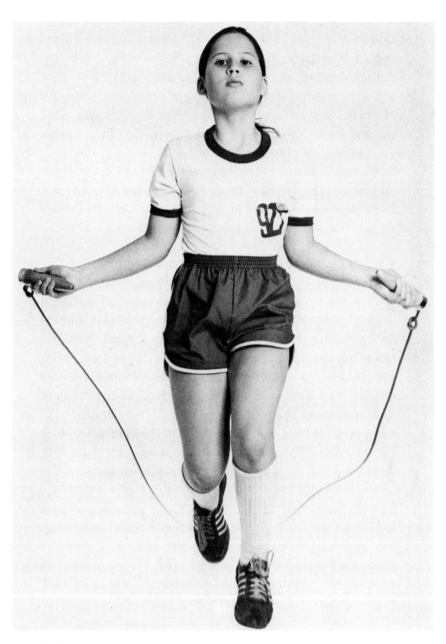

S. "Totes" Carney shows us
her running step

## Jump to Music

Put on a record and start perfecting the running step. Your arms must remain stationary as the rope turns: you just move your wrists. This wrist action is going to tone your upper arms, chest, and back. You're using all those muscles, even though you're keeping the arms as still as possible.

Run in place over the rope, knees high: right foot, left, right. Keep practicing; you'll have the technique perfected in no time.

Here are some common problems my students experience when they begin to learn the running step, and the solutions:

• Bouncing between steps. This is actually another step that you'll learn later. Right now, concentrate on eliminating that bounce. Go back to practicing the step, holding the rope in front of you with both hands. Do the step in slow motion until you have the rhythm back, then try it again while you jump over the rope.

• Single footing. This is when the same foot comes forward for each step instead of changing. Go back to practicing in slow motion, as above.

• Running forward. If you can't stay in the same place, pick a mark on the floor or put a string or tape marker on your carpet and stay on it as you jump. Think of jumping up, not forward.

• Jumping too hard. Turn off your music and listen to your feet touch the floor. There should be no sound, as if your feet are autumn leaves touching the ground. If you are pounding down, you're not jumping correctly. If you live in an apartment, your downstairs neighbor will not be pleased. Jumping too hard can damage your joints, the small bones of your feet, and such. The proper shoes are essential for cushioning your feet as they touch the floor. REMEMBER: jumping is touching off, *not* landing.

JUMP for another minute. Concentrate on keeping your arms in the proper position. Make sure that only the wrists are turning the rope. Arms remain still. Breathe through your nose only. If you breathe through your mouth, you will tire yourself out much faster.

Now, exhale, bend over, and do a deep, RESTING STRETCH. When you feel collected, come up. It's time to learn another step, one that you'll always enjoy and come back to, no matter how many other steps you master. Go on to this next step, even if you haven't mastered the running step. The comparison will help you when you go back to the running step.

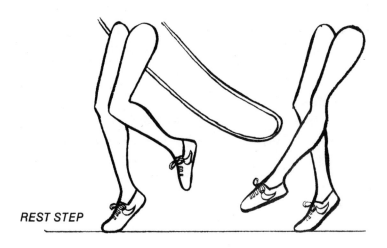

REST STEP

## The Rest Step

Jump over the rope, landing on the ball of your right foot. As the rope is turning over your head, bounce again on your right foot with a little hop (or skip), kicking the left foot out a bit.

Jump over the rope, landing on the ball of your left foot, with a hop (or skip) as your right foot kicks out.

Alternate feet, each time jumping onto the ball of the foot and taking a little skip: jump and skip on the right foot, jump and skip on the left foot.

This is called the rest step because you are allowed an extra beat (or bounce) between jumps. You jump twice on each foot: jump and rest, jump and rest. This allows you to slow your breathing down. The rest step is like slow jogging, as opposed to a full-out run. Once you become used to this step, you'll be amazed to find that you can actually rest and relax while jumping.

Breathe through your nose only, as with all other steps. Relax your legs as well. As you get into the rhythm, you'll notice that the back leg will naturally drift forward on the extra beat, in order to be in place to go over the rope.

Practice this step first with the rope held in front of you. Relax: jump and rest.

You will use the rest step to warm up at the beginning of your workout every day and to relax between the more strenuous steps.

## Jump to Music

Put on a record, and jump! Work on the rest step until you feel you have the rhythm. Then go back and do the running step for a count of twenty times over the rope. Next, the rest step twenty times. Keep alternating until you are tired, then bend over into the resting stretch and relax.

Now you're going to finish up with one extra exercise.

## Leg Raises

It's time for a little concentrated exercise. The only area jumping rope doesn't reshape is the midsection, so for total shaping I recommend leg raises to supplement your rope-jumping program. (WARNING: do *not* attempt this exercise if you have impaired circulation or heart or back problems.)

Lie on your back on a rug, a large towel, or an exercise mat. Place your hands, palms down, *under your buttocks*. Raise your head off the floor, tucking your chin close to your chest. Keep your head in this position throughout the exercise. This is a *must*; it keeps strain off the lower back.

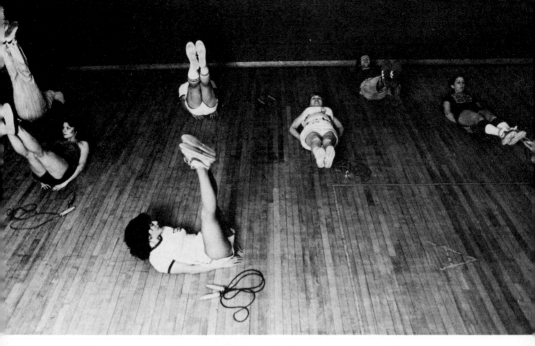

*Leg raises are great for your waist and abdominals*

Raise your legs, knees locked, off the floor. Breathe naturally, keep the knees straight, and bring the legs to a ninety-degree angle. Then lower your legs to about an inch off the floor, making sure your heels do not touch the floor.

Repeat until you have counted out ten leg raises. Lower your legs and feet *gently* to the floor. Relax, arms at your sides. Take several slow, deep breaths: inhale through your nose, exhale through your mouth.

Now, get back into position—palms under buttocks, head up (chin to chest). Do ten more leg raises, breathing naturally. Some people inhale as they raise their legs and exhale as they lower them—or vice versa. It doesn't matter so long as you breathe in a steady rhythm. Never hold your breath.

*Note:* If you are eager to really trim down your middle as quickly as possible, attach ankle weights to each ankle before doing your leg raises. Ankle weights are available at sporting-goods stores for about nine to thirteen dollars. They come in two-, two-and-a-half-, and three-pound sizes. The heavier the weight, the faster the results. When you want to shape up a muscle that has been neglected, you have to be prepared to work.

### Today's Last Word

After this first session, your muscles are going to hurt. You'll feel them tomorrow. Even if you are in generally good condition, you have just used muscles, both in the jumping and the leg raises, that haven't been worked in a long time. I guarantee that you will experience some soreness, perhaps a lot.

As soon as possible after your workout, rub your calves with liniment. Massage your legs really hard—try to get down to the bone. If you can take a sauna or steam bath the same day as the workout, great. If not, soak in a relaxing, hot tub as soon as you can. Rub your calves again before bedtime.

Don't let calf pain stop you from jumping rope tomorrow, no matter how much soreness you feel. The aches will go away in a couple of days, and they won't come back. Don't get mad at me and stomp on this book. Get mad at yourself for being in poor shape, and cheer up because you've started to do something about it.

That's all for today. Go rub your muscles, or use a comfrey poultice.

### DAY #2

No matter how sore your muscles feel today, you should work out. Don't lose momentum now that you've started jumping into shape. Besides, after you get warmed up and into the rhythm of jumping, you'll practically forget all those aches. Notice the halo forming around your head because you're so spunky and conscientious. Let's go to it.

### Warm-Up Review—Practice Without Music

Just to get into the rhythm, hold your rope in front of you and practice the steps you learned yesterday in slow motion: the *running step* and the *rest step*. Today you're going to begin trying to perfect those steps, jumping with a smooth transition from one to the other.

When you do the running step you should have the feeling that you're prancing like a pony. Don't forget to breathe through your nose only. Check your form when you start jumping over the rope. Make sure that your arms are in proper position; don't let them slip below your waist. In order to have a good workout you must have good form. Turn the rope with your wrists only. You are the center of a perfect, moving circle.

### Jump to Music: 15 minutes

Don't worry—you're not going to be jumping for the entire time. I want you to jump until you get tired, then go into your resting stretch. I'd like you to alternate between the two steps: twenty-five *running steps,* fifty *rest steps,* back and forth. If you trip over the rope and have trouble getting your rhythm, don't become discouraged! Try to keep jumping or dancing while you get the rope back into starting position.

If you seem to be having a lot of trouble, go back to doing the steps with the rope held in front of you. Jumping rope isn't as easy as it looks. You're mastering a new exercise, one that's going to get you in super shape. You have to expect it to be hard work as well as fun. Keep your mind focused on the results: your firmer, shapelier figure, your improved circulation and breathing control. You're jumping your way to a new you!

### Leg Raises

Now you've jumped and stretched for fifteen minutes. Congratulations! You've overcome those sore muscles. Let's finish the workout by zeroing in on those stomach muscles. Do two sets of ten leg raises, resting between sets. Keep your palms placed under your buttocks, head up, chin on chest. Keep your knees straight and lower your heels to just an inch off of the floor. After you've finished both sets, rest. Close your eyes, let your arms lie by your sides. Breathe deeply in through your nose, exhale through your mouth.

You've completed your second day. Rub your muscles again with liniment and take a nice, hot bath.

### DAY #3

Your muscles may still feel a little sore, but it will be over soon. Once those aches go away, they're gone for good.

### Warm-Up Review—Practice Without Music

Make sure you have a firm grip on the rope handles. Check your form as you jump: keep those arms up at waist level. Pretend you're a feather, and think of making no noise as the balls of your feet gently touch the floor. Don't exhaust your breathing system: breathe through the nose only. Practice perfecting a smooth transition between steps: the running step and the rest step.

### Jump to Music: 5 minutes

Do twenty-five *running steps*, fifty *rest steps*, and repeat the cycle until you get tired. Then bend over into a deep *stretch*. After you're rested, start jumping again. Practice in slow motion, without the rope, if you're having trouble. Now, turn off the music; it's time to learn a new step.

### Doubles Step

Jump, jump, jump, straight over the rope with *both feet*

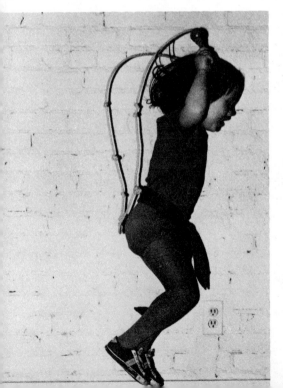

*India displays
her doubles and proves that
you can start
jumping at any age*

landing on the balls of the feet only. Keep the knees bent to absorb the shock. Jump over the rope each time it hits the floor: no bounces in between jumps.

Practice the step before you jump over the rope. Concentrate on coming down on the balls of your feet as lightly as possible. Listen to yourself. Sneakers come down heavier than running shoes; whichever you're wearing, don't pound.

### Jump to Music: 5 minutes

Now you've got three steps: your *rest step*, the *running step*, and *doubles*. Pretty soon you're going to have all kinds of steps to do, and jumping rope will become more and more fun. You'll be dancing on the rope in no time. Perfecting a lot of steps takes away the boredom of repetition. You'll go from one step to another, using the rest step to slow down your breathing when you get tired. When you stop jumping, go into the resting stretch position to collect yourself.

### Leg Raises

Lie down on the floor and go into the proper position. Do two sets of ten leg raises, resting in between. When you've finished, close your eyes and rest a few more minutes, breathing deeply in through your nose, out through your mouth.

You've just completed your third day. Rub your muscles again, and take a sauna or hot bath.

### DAY #4

Let's get into it right away.

### Warm-Up Review—Practice Without Music

Review your *running step*, *rest step*, and *doubles*. Any time you have problems with a step, go back to doing it in slow motion, holding your rope in front of you. Work on your form and make a smooth transition when changing from one step to another. Before you begin your workout to music, here's another step.

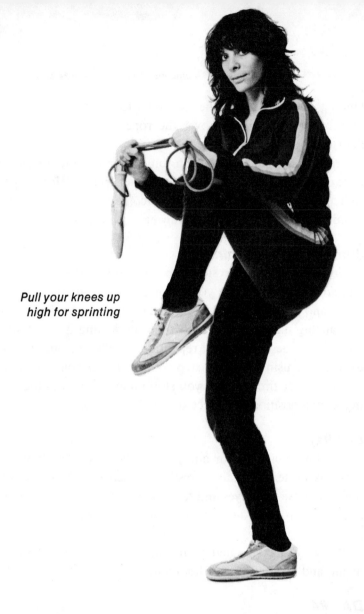

*Pull your knees up
high for sprinting*

### Sprinting Step

This is a variation of the *running step*. Run in place, over
the rope, *bringing your knees up* as high as you can.

Jump over the rope with your right foot, knees high.

Jump over the rope with your left foot, knees high. Do not
bounce in between steps.

Sprint for speed, to build up your leg muscles. Stay on your
toes, and keep your knees up!

Practice the step in slow motion, in the practice position, until you have the rhythm of it. This step will give you a good workout.

### Jump to Music: 15 minutes

Jump, alternating the four steps you've learned, until you're tired, and then go into the deep resting stretch. Work on changing smoothly from step to step. Do twenty-five *running steps*, fifty *rest steps*, twenty-five *doubles*, fifty *rest steps*, ten *sprinting steps*, fifty *rest steps*, and so forth.

Try to become part of the music. Turn the volume higher than you would usually have it for background listening. Let the music take you over your jump rope. Really respond to those rhythms, and think about what good shape you're getting into. Stretch when you become tired, then return to your rope dancing.

### Leg Raises

Today, because you have a lot more stamina now than you did when you began, do two sets of fifteen leg raises. Remember to breathe naturally. Rest in between sets and when you're finished. Close your eyes and imagine your firmer, slimmer body. Take deep breaths, exhaling through your mouth.

Your muscles may still ache a little, but maybe not. If they do, keep up the liniment rubs. Be proud of yourself. You're learning to have a disciplined workout. That's what jumping rope is: an exercise that you can do everyday to establish your own self-discipline. Even as it becomes more and more fun, you have to be serious about it.

Getting into shape—and staying that way for the rest of your life—requires self-discipline. Even on those days when you feel rotten, tired, or depressed, you have to force yourself to spend those fifteen minutes on your body. Once you've done it, you'll feel better mentally, as well as physically, for having made yourself do it. Exercise brings up your energy level, and it makes you feel good all over.

## DAY #5

### Warm-up Review—Practice with Music

Go over all the steps you've learned so far: the *running step*, *rest step*, *doubles*, and the *sprinting step*. Work on having perfect form. Breathe through your nose. Today, you're going to add a new step to your fast-growing repertoire.

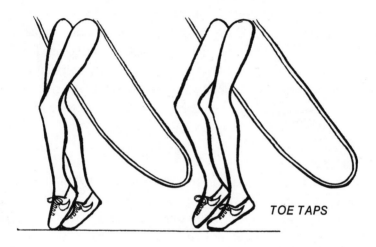

TOE TAPS

### Toe Taps

Jump onto the ball of the right foot, your left toe tapping alongside of your right foot.

Jump onto the ball of your left foot, tapping the right toe alongside of the left foot.

Keep alternating feet. Make sure that one toe taps simultaneously as the ball of the other foot touches the floor.

Toe taps usually become a favorite step of my students and have long been the professional boxer's best long-term workout step.

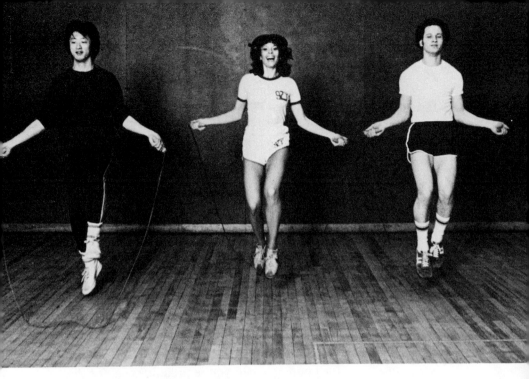

*Sidney and Michael (right) tapping toes*
*as Jason does a running step*

Let's practice, holding your rope in front of you. Toe taps mainly involve a shift of weight. You stay in the same spot. Jump in place, feet close together. With each jump, shift your weight from one foot to the other, tapping the toe of the opposite foot on the floor at the same time.

While you're learning, you must concentrate on one step at a time. Once you've mastered a new step, you work on adding it to the others so you can jump continuously and make a clean transition (no tripping) from one step to another.

### Jump to Music: 15 minutes

Work on perfecting your *toe taps* first. Then alternate them with the other steps: twenty-five *toe taps*, fifty *rest steps*, twenty-five *running steps*, fifty *rest steps*, ten *sprinting steps*, fifty *rest steps*, twenty-five *doubles*, and so on.

When you're tired, go into your resting stretch. And today, you're going to learn another stretch.

### Open Leg Stretch

Sit on the floor, legs opened out as far to the sides as you can get them. Flex your feet, toes pointed upward, and keep the back of your knees flat on the floor, legs straight.

Sit up straight, don't round your back. Tilt your groin area into the floor. Now lean forward, as far as you can go, chest to floor. Breathe evenly, in through the nose, out through the mouth. Stay there—don't come up, and don't bounce in this position.

Eventually you *will* be able to place your chest on the floor: that's your goal and everyone should be able to stretch that way. Don't take deep breaths into your stomach—maintain shallow chest breathing.

This stretch is to be used the same way as the standing stretch —as a substitute for jumping when you're tired. I repeat for the umpteenth time: when you're not jumping you *must* stretch, so you will get a complete fifteen-minute workout.

*Your body will be this stretched— you can do it!*

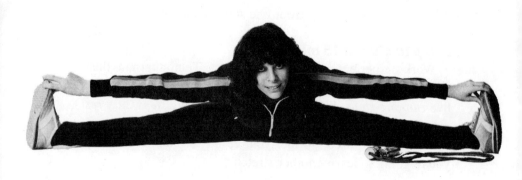

### Leg Raises

Today you're going to repeat your two sets of fifteen leg raises, resting in between sets for a minute, and afterward, taking deep breaths.

Now, I'm going to introduce you to a slogan taught to me by martial arts Grand Master Peter Urban. The words have inspired me for many years and have become my motto of self-discipline. I hope they will help you, too. LET'S GO! KEEP GOING! THERE *IS* NOTHING ELSE! Think it to yourself, say it out loud, use this slogan when you need a boost to keep on going. I'll have a lot more to say about self-discipline later on, in chapter eight. Turn to it now, and read it many times during the next nine days.

### DAY #6

This is going to be a review day. You will do your timed jumping and stretching to music, working on the smooth transition from step to step. Try to keep in a pattern, alternating all the steps you've learned so far: the *running step, rest step, doubles, the sprinting step* (make yourself do this one fifteen times in a row), and *toe taps*. Listen to the music, really allow yourself to get into the rhythms of it. Don't neglect your form: hands firmly gripping the handles, arms in proper position, wrists only turning the rope, breathing through the nose only. LET'S GO! KEEP GOING! THERE *IS* NOTHING ELSE!

### Jump to Music: 15 minutes

Jump! Switch smoothly from step to step. When you get tired, stretch. Use the open leg floor stretch: legs open wide, feet flexed, backs of knees flat on floor. Lean forward with chest as close as possible to the floor. Don't bounce. Shallow breathing: in through your nose, out through your mouth.

### Leg Raises

Again, today, two sets of fifteen, resting in between. Don't ever do these leg raises without placing your hands, palms down, under your buttocks and bringing your head up with chin to your chest. This is a must; it keeps all strain off of your lower back. Now rest, and totally relax yourself.

Almost all beginners experience varying degrees of regression at some point while they're learning. Usually it manifests itself in the form of continuous tripping over the rope, or getting tangled up. Sometimes it happens early in the training, sometimes later. It may never happen at all, but if it does *don't worry about it*. Everything will come together sooner or later. You just have to keep at it and return to working in slow motion without the rope. Keep your mind focused ahead to the benefits you are reaping from getting in shape. There is no doubt about it: when your body is fit, you are going to feel good about yourself. This inner confidence is going to carry over into every area of your life. Your friends and family will see a positive change in you. You will be able to look into the mirror and smile.

## DAY #7

Today you will learn a couple of new steps. Let's work on them first, and then assimilate them into your rope routine with music.

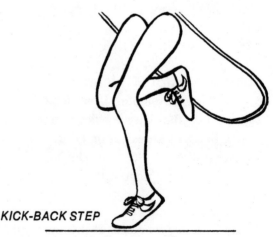

**KICK-BACK STEP**

## Kick-Back Step

This is another variation of the old standby, the running step. For this step, you run over the rope, alternating feet with each jump—no bounces in between. As you step over the rope, kick the heel up toward your buttocks. In doing this you are more likely to catch the rope: don't let your heel go out away from the body. Bring it *up*, and you won't get tangled.

Hold your rope in front of you and practice in slow motion. Try to lift your heel up to your buttocks, as high as you can. Think of lifting the heel up, rather than pushing it back. This step is excellent for toning your buttocks and upper thighs.

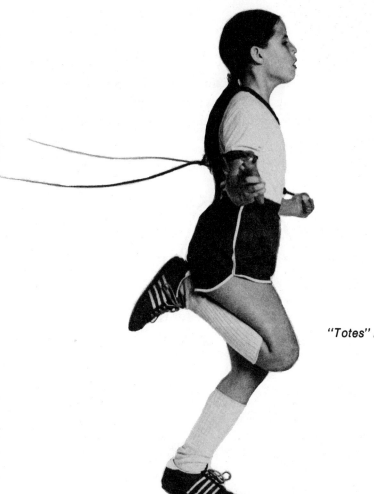

*"Totes" kicks back*

The two versions of the running step—the kick-back and sprinting steps—are ways to add spot shaping to your jumping routine. When you want to work your buttocks, you can concentrate on doing the kick-back. If you're eager to dissolve those lumpy front thighs, then do the running step, adding as many sprints as you can manage.

Being able to control your feet in the kick-back step, pulling the heel toward the buttock, is the same kind of feeling you get with the open leg stretch when you flex your toes back toward you. Keep practicing the kick-back step without the rope until you feel you have mastered it. Now try it with the rope.

Before you put on the music, here is another step.

### Side-to-Side Step

To get the rhythm of this step, go back to toe taps, and practice them.

Now, spread out the toe taps. Jump from right foot to left foot (on your toes), going from side to side, jumping over an imaginary line. The pacing is just like the toe taps, only you're spreading your space.

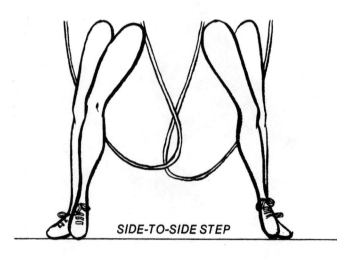

SIDE-TO-SIDE STEP

Practice your side-to-side step with the rope. Turn the rope with your wrists only. Keep your upper body still. This step teaches you how to go from one spot to another quickly. Once you've mastered it, you will know how to avoid things coming at you—you will be able to get out of the way fast. This step builds timing.

### Jump to Music: 15 minutes

First, practice the two new steps to music: *the kick-back step* and *the side-to-side step*. When you feel you've got them down, then jump to the rhythm of the music, alternating all the steps you've learned so far: *running step, rest step, doubles, toe taps, sprinting step* (don't neglect this one), *kick-back,* and *side-to-side step*. Dance to the music.

Stretch whenever you feel tired, but today you will transfer all your stretching to the floor. Do only the open leg stretching.

### Leg Raises

Do two sets of fifteen, resting in between and afterward. Your whole midsection should be firming up nicely by now. Aren't you glad you've stuck with it?

### DAY #8

Today will be another review day. So far you have learned seven rope-jumping routines. These will improve your coordination, your heart, and your shape. These are the basics, and all sorts of new steps and variations are yet to come. Later on, you'll probably be inventing your own steps. (Write me and let me know what they are: you may invent something completely new.) The point of learning all these routines is to give you versatility on the rope and to take the boredom out of exercise. As you become an expert jumper, your friends will probably urge you to show them how. Before you know it, you may become a teacher like me. A person can meet a lot of new friends by jumping rope. You just wait and see.

## Jump to Music: 15 minutes

Review all the steps you have learned so far: *running step, rest step, doubles, toe taps, sprinting step, kick-back, and side-to-side step.* Concentrate on your perfect form and the change-over from one step to another. Build up your repetitions: do fifty steps where you were doing twenty-five before and a hundred rest steps when you want to quiet down your breathing. You're building your stamina. You're getting into great shape!

Remember: LET'S GO! KEEP GOING! THERE *IS* NOTHING ELSE! And here is another of Master Peter Urban's slogans for you: *Plan your work, work your plan.*

Alternate the jumping with *open leg stretches* on the floor. Here is another floor stretch for you.

## Closed Leg Stretches

Sit on the floor, back straight, legs together. Flex your feet, toes pointing upward. Keep the backs of your knees flat on the floor.

Bend over, chest to knees, elbows and forearms resting on floor on either sides of the legs. Your goal is to rest your elbows and forearms on the floor while doing this stretch.

Don't bounce. Once you are in this stretch, don't come up: stay there for at least a count of twenty-five.

## Leg Raises

Do two sets of fifteen leg raises, resting in between and afterward, relaxing totally.

## DAY #9

Today you will learn a new step, an easy one.

## The Two-step

Jump over the rope twice on each foot before changing feet. Jump onto the ball of the right foot. Repeat right.

Jump onto the ball of the left foot. Repeat left.

Alternate, jumping right, right, left, left, and so on.

I call this my rhythm step; it's great with music. Practice in slow motion, holding your rope in front of you. Then try it with the rope.

### Jump to Music: 15 minutes

Today I have another quote to spur you on, again from Master Peter Urban: *Winners never quit, quitters never win.*

From here on, you can stop counting the repetitions of the steps. (This is optional; some jumpers *like* to count the number of repetitions for each step they do. There are even digital jump ropes that will do the counting for you.)

Jump and dance to the music, alternating your steps at whim. Force yourself to do the *sprinting step* from time to time, at least fifteen times in a row when you do it. Get into the rhythm of the music, and jump rope to your various steps: *running, rest step, doubles, toe taps, sprinting step, kick-back, side-to-side step,* and the new *two-step.*

Stretch when you're not jumping: both the *open leg* stretches and the *closed leg* stretches.

### Leg Raises

Do two sets of fifteen leg raises, resting in between and afterward.

Aren't you proud of yourself? You've just finished your ninth day.

### DAY #10

As a special treat for today, you're going to learn another new step, with two variations.

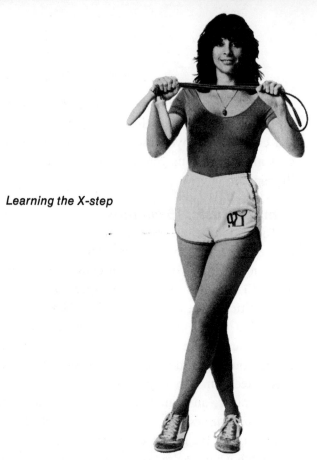

*Learning the X-step*

## The X-Step

This step is named after the cross your feet make each time you jump.

Jump, crossing your right foot in front of your left. Jump with both feet open.

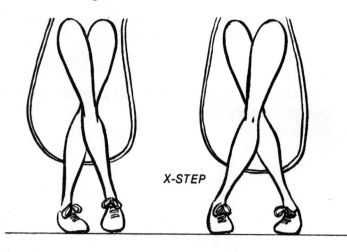

X-STEP

Jump, crossing your left foot in front of your right. Jump with both feet open.

Stay way up on your toes. Don't bounce between jumps. Jump, crossing right. Jump open. Jump, crossing left. Alternate.

As always when learning a new step, practice in slow motion with your rope held out in front of you. Then try it with the rope.

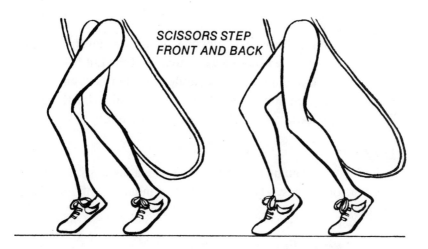

SCISSORS STEP
FRONT AND BACK

## The Scissors Step—Front & Back

In this step, you move your feet alternately forward and backward.

Jump, landing on the balls of the feet: right foot forward, left foot back.

Jump, landing on the balls of the feet: left foot forward, right foot back.

Alternate feet.

Practice this step like all the others, first without the rope, then with the rope.

## Jump to Music: 15 minutes

First of all, work on the *X-step* and the *front-back step*. Then incorporate these two new routines into the ones you already know. Jump, practicing all of them: *running, rest step, doubles, toe taps, sprinting step, kick-back, side-to-side step, two-step, X-step,* and *scissors step.*

Concentrate, as always, on perfecting your form, and maintaining a smooth transition between steps. Listen to the music, and move with it. By now you should really be dancing on that rope.

When you're tired, go into your *open leg stretches* and *closed leg stretches.*

### Leg Raises

Today, you only have to do one set of leg raises, but do *twenty* nonstop. Keep those legs straight and the knees locked. Make sure your palms are resting under your buttocks and your head is resting on your chest. Now, relax totally, breathing in through your nose and out through your mouth.

### DAY #11

Today you're going to learn how to take a break while jumping, via rope tricks. The rope is worked independently of your jumping.

### Rope Twirls—Figure Eights

Jump rope, using any of the steps you know. Stop dead in your tracks and, still keeping the rope moving to the beat of the music, grasp the rope handles with both hands held in front of you.

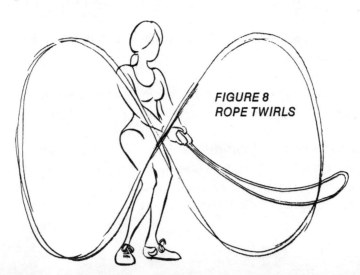

FIGURE 8
ROPE TWIRLS

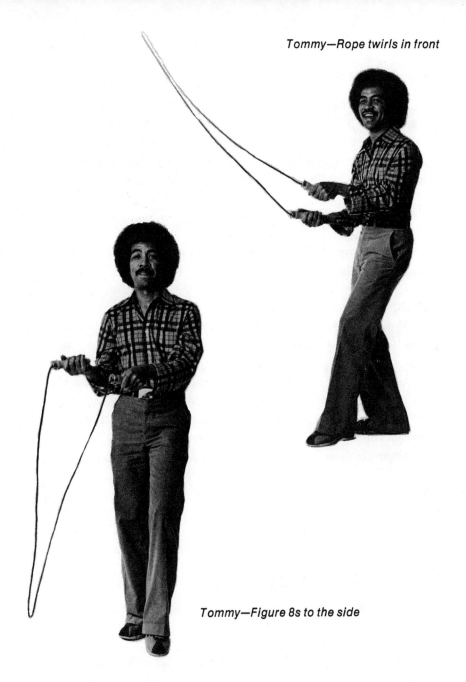

*Tommy—Rope twirls in front*

*Tommy—Figure 8s to the side*

Make figure eights with the rope, striking the floor directly in front of you. Do this to the rhythm of the music.

Without breaking the rhythm, open the rope handles and start jumping again. When you can do this without breaking rhythm, your coordination gets an A-plus.

These figure eights with the rope may also be done while you continue to jump in any step you wish. Just hit the floor with the rope as you jump, making sure it's right in front of you so you don't strike yourself. Then open the rope and go back to jumping over it. This is a great step for showing off!

### Rope Twirls—One-handed

Jump rope in any step. Stop and hold the rope handles in one hand. Turn the rope in circles at your side, standing still or jumping in place as you twirl the rope.

### Jump to Music: 15 minutes

As always, work on perfecting your snappy transition from step to step: *running step, rest step, doubles, toe taps, sprinting step* (do these for a count of twenty), *kick-back, side-to-side step, two-step, X-step,* and *scissors step.* Then, from time to time, stop in your tracks, and work on one or both of the *rope twirls.* Continue jumping the next time you work the rope twirls. Variety is the spice of life and jumping rope.

Alternate your jumping with the *open leg stretches* and the *closed leg stretches.* By now, however, your stamina should have improved so much that your jumping time greatly outdistances your stretching time.

LET'S GO! KEEP GOING! THERE *IS* NOTHING ELSE!

### Leg Raises

Today, do two sets of twenty leg raises, with a good rest in between and afterward. Your mirror image is improving day by day, and you must be pleased with your progress. Exercise helps you make the most out of every day. Jumping rope is one of the most enjoyable aerobic exercises—it keeps your body in shape as well as your heart.

### DAY #12

Here's another fancy step for your jumping pleasure. It's a show-off step, and you'll love it.

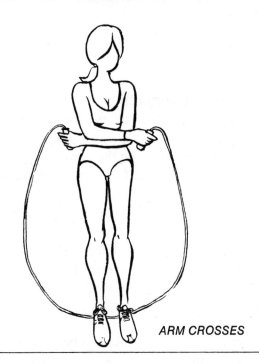

ARM CROSSES

## Arm Crosses

Jump rope in any step. For practice, use the *doubles step* or *toe taps*. Jump rhythmically.

Cross your arms evenly at the forearms on the downward swing of the rope, and jump through the loop that has formed in front of your body. Make sure your rope hits the ground. Keep your knees bent.

Uncross your arms for the next swing of the rope.

Practice the arm crosses with the rope. Watch that you don't cross your arms at the wrists or you won't have enough space to jump through.

This showy move doesn't have to be constant. You can jump several times, then cross your arms and jump through the rope. Then return to normal jumping. You are at liberty to do the arm crosses as often or infrequently as you like. You will impress all who witness this marvelous display of coordination and jazzy jumping.

If you have problems with the arm crosses, concentrate on hitting the ground with the rope every time you cross your arms. Stick with it; it'll come.

### Jump to Music: 15 minutes

Jump, jump, jump! *Running step, rest step, doubles, toe taps, sprinting step, kick-back, side-to-side step, two-step, X-step,* and *scissors step.* Work on the *arm crosses.* Stop and do a display of *rope twirls.* Change from step to step smoothly. Turn the rope with your wrists only. Make sure your arms are up at your waist. Breathe through your nose. Look forward, and think *up!*

Rest with the *open* and *closed leg stretches.* You should be able to stretch really deeply by now. If you aren't, you must not be pushing yourself enough. Work on those stretches.

### Leg Raises

Do twenty leg raises, twice. Rest in between and afterward. Your middle is getting a real workout. If you are exceptionally thick around the middle, you should do a hundred leg raises a day—in sets of ten, twenty, whatever is best for you.

The leg raises should be kept up at least three times a week as a maintenance after you have completed the fourteen-day shape-up program.

### DAY #13

By now you should have developed your favorite jumping steps, ones you like doing better than others. That's fine. But make sure you always get in a few sets of the sprinting step, to give your heart a good workout. And keep in practice with all the steps: you'll find that you'll change favorites from time to time. After this chapter you will find additional fancy steps to add when you feel like it. Try to work on a new step as often as possible—don't get in a jump-rope rut. Here is today's entry for your jumping variety.

### Backward Steps

Most of the steps you know can be done backward.

Start with the rope in front of your feet. Swing it up over your head and jump backward as the rope passes underneath your feet.

Some people have a natural affinity for backward jumping and can do all the steps they know easily. Others never get the hang of it for more than a few jumps. It doesn't matter. Try jumping backward with your rope, and see whether this is going to be your cup of tea.

### Jump to Music: 15 minutes

Jump backward, jump forward! Do all the steps, in whatever succession pleases you: *running, rest step, doubles, toe taps, sprinting step, kick-back, side-to-side step, two-step, X-step, scissors step, arm crosses, rope twirls.*

And here's another slogan to keep you going, also from Master Urban: *Discipline equals freedom.* LET'S GO! KEEP GOING! THERE *IS* NOTHING ELSE! And have a really good time!

### Open and Closed Leg Stretches

Don't forget your *open* and *closed leg stretches.* Work on achieving the optimum stretch. Always try to stretch farther; don't ever slack off. Concentrate on relaxing your muscles as you stretch. Breathe evenly, in through your nose, out through your mouth. Don't ever bounce when you're stretching.

### Leg Raises

Do two sets of twenty, resting in between and afterward. You have just completed your thirteenth day. Congratulations!

### DAY #14

You've reached your fourteenth day. You can see for yourself that it's been worth it. By now, your stamina will be greatly improved, your figure will be more toned and lithe. In short, you should be feeling terrific about yourself. Today there are no new steps to learn, just a review of the past two weeks. Go to it!

### Jump to Music: 15 minutes

This time, you're going to jump for the full fifteen minutes, going from one step to another: the *running step, rest step, doubles, toe taps, sprinting step, kick-back step, side-to-side step, two-step, X-step, scissors step, arm crosses, backward steps.* Stop and work on your *rope twirls* while you stand still or jump in place. You've built up your energy enormously in the past two weeks. You should be able to jump and dance on the rope for the entire time without having to collapse into a resting stretch. Jumping for fifteen minutes straight is no hardship—it's really very little.

The music you use today should have a good fast beat. Your jumping should really be a dancing workout. Let  the music carry your feet over the rope.

### Open and Closed Leg Stretches

After you've finished your fifteen-minute jump, get down on the floor and do both the open and closed leg stretches. Really stretch those muscles: you should be able to do deep stretches by now.

### Leg Raises

Because it's graduation day, you get to do three sets of twenty leg raises. Be sure to rest in between sets and afterward. Totally relax. Breathe in through your nose, out through your mouth, and close your eyes.

### MAINTENANCE PROGRAM

Now that you're in shape, stay that way! Don't backslide. You've worked hard to get to this point, and you're going to have to keep it up to maintain your health and energy. Maintenance means exercising for the rest of your life. To really benefit from exercise, you have to do it and keep on doing it. Pretty soon, you'll be so hooked that you won't be able to stand *not* doing it.

Your maintenance program requires you to exercise for fifteen to thirty minutes, a minimum of *three times a week.* (Don't let more than two days elapse between workouts.)

Jump rope for fifteen minutes, then go into your *open* and *closed leg stretches* and *leg raises* to cool you down slowly.

Or, alternate your rope jumping with any other good aerobic exercise: walking at a forced pace, jogging, running, swimming, cycling (on a bike or stationary cycle), running in place, bench stepping or stair climbing (continuous running up and down flights of stairs). You'll find books on other aerobic exercises listed in the Bibliography. Some days you may feel like jumping rope; other days you might want to swim. It doesn't matter what you do, as long as you do it faithfully and conscientiously.

Now you know how to have a disciplined, rope-jumping workout. Make jumping rope part of your permanent exercise repertoire: enjoy it for the rest of your life. In the next chapter, you will find some additional fancy steps and routines to learn and enjoy. Jump on the rope! Skip on the rope! Dance on the rope! And stay with it. Once you're in shape, don't lose it. LET'S GO! KEEP GOING! THERE *IS* NOTHING ELSE!

# Chapter 4

# Rope Dancing: Fancy Steps and Jumping Games

By now, you know for yourself that music is everything. Jumping to fast melodies turns into rope dancing—gliding from step to step, inventing your own routines, having fun on the rope. The more you jump, the more new steps and rope patterns you'll invent for yourself.

Just in case you need some ideas, here are some additional steps to spur you on. For learning these, the same basic rules apply. First, practice each new step in slow motion, holding the rope in front of you. Once you feel you have developed the rhythm of the step, start jumping. Remember the following basic rules (I can't repeat these often enough!):

- Don't pound the floor. Jump gently on the balls of the feet only.
- Always keep your knees bent.
- Breathe through your nose only.
- Wrists only for turning the rope. Keep arms still.

## FANCY STEPS FOR FUN

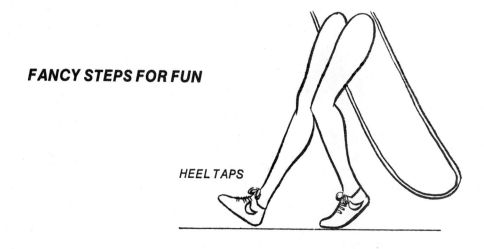

*HEEL TAPS*

### Heel Taps

Jump onto the ball of your right foot. Simultaneously, tap your left heel on the floor out in front of you.

Jump onto the ball of your left foot. At the same time, tap your right heel out in front of you.

Continue, alternating feet. Be sure that you don't put any weight on your heel as you come down.

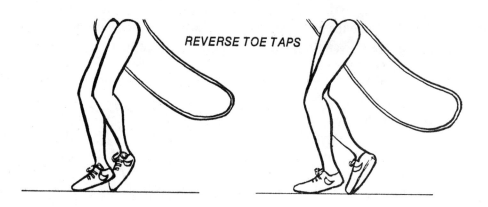

*REVERSE TOE TAPS*

### Reverse Toe Taps

Jump onto the ball of your right foot. At the same time, tap your left toe on the floor, just behind your right foot.

Jump onto the ball of your left foot, while you tap your right toe on the floor behind you.

Continue, alternating feet.

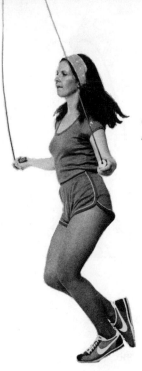

*Claudia flies through reverse toe taps*

### Side Taps

Jump onto the ball of your right foot. Simultaneously, fling your left leg to the side and tap the left toe on the floor.

Jump onto the ball of your left foot, while you fling your right leg to the side and tap with the toe of your right foot.

Alternate feet.

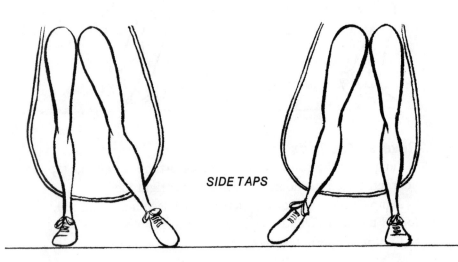

SIDE TAPS

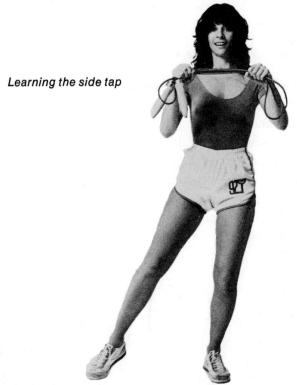

*Learning the side tap*

### The "Dancer" Step

Spring up off the floor. Land on the balls of both feet, with the toes turned in and the heels turned out. Let the knees touch on this inward turn.

Land on the balls of the feet, with toes turned out and heels turned in. Keep the knees bent outward.

Continue, alternating, toes in, toes out.

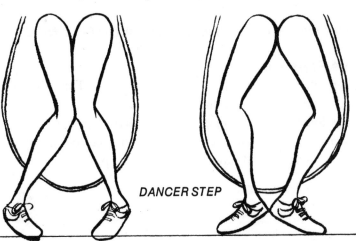

DANCER STEP

### Kick-back Crossovers

Land on the ball of your right foot. Kick your left leg back behind the right leg.

Land on the ball of your left foot. Kick your right leg back behind your left leg.

Continue, alternating. Be sure to keep knees well bent. You'll find, as you get into the rhythm of the step, that you'll experience a natural weight shift that will have you bending slightly at the waist.

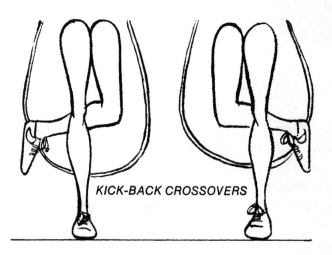

KICK-BACK CROSSOVERS

## STEPS FOR THOSE WHO ENJOY A CHALLENGE

### Double Rope Turns

Do two turns of the rope for every one jump. This will require a higher jump and a slight body tuck.

Impossible? The *Guinness Book of World Records* lists Katsuma Suzuki of Japan as the record holder for multiple turns. He managed to do five turns in one jump!

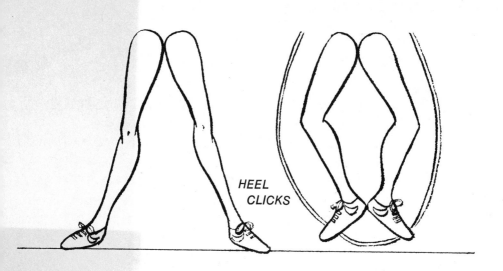

HEEL
CLICKS

## Heel Clicks

Begin with your feet spread apart.
Spring up, clicking your heels together.
Land on the balls of both feet, with feet spread apart.
Continue, alternating heel clicks and foot spreads.

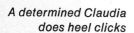

*A determined Claudia
does heel clicks*

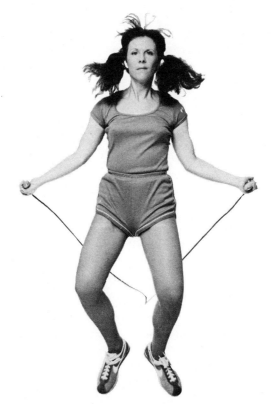

### Jog 'n Jump

Take your rope out to the running track, and jump and run or jog at the same time. Basically, this is just your *running step* —instead of running in place you're out to cover as much distance as possible.

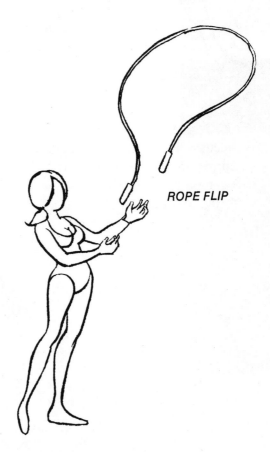

ROPE FLIP

### Rope Flips

This is another variation of the rope twirls.

Toss the rope up into the air as you release the rope handles. This causes the rope to make one revolution. Regrasp the rope handles when the rope comes back down.

Be sure to practice this outside or where you have lots of room. Keep people away from your practice area for safety.

## MAKING UP NEW STEPS

Rope jumping never has to become monotonous or boring. With all of the variations you now know, you should be able to come up with many new combinations of steps—flings, twirls, kicks, taps, front, back, and sideways. There are dozens of routines to be invented, many of them based on steps you know already. Try new steps and if you like them and they feel good, add them to your permanent repertoire.

## JUMPING GAMES FOR TWO OR MORE

Now I will touch on the kinds of rope-jumping antics you remember (or may have forgotten) from childhood. Not that these games are only for kids: you may enjoy some or all of them. These are games for fun, and they will not take the place of your daily workout. Nevertheless, it's good to know them. They're terrific for your coordination. Some of the see-how-long-you-can-jump ones are stamina building.    These games require long ropes—#10 sash cord is fine. (For additional books on rope games, see Bibliography.)

*Group games are fun*

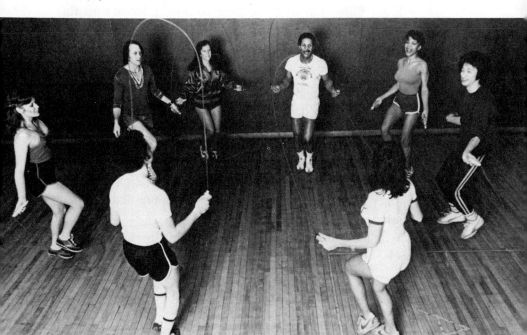

### Side-by-side Together

You and your partner must stand side by side, facing the same direction. You turn the rope with your right hand, your partner turns it with his or her left hand. Jump together, forward or backward. To make it more difficult, you can face one direction, while your partner faces the other.

### Jumping In

One player turns the rope and jumps. The second player jumps in, facing the first jumper. The two players jump together for awhile, and then the second player jumps out, leaving space for another player to jump in.

### Jumping In with Enders

"Enders" are the two people who hold either end of a long rope, while one or more players jump in. Once in, the jumper jumps to any one of hundreds of jumping rhymes. When the jumper misses he or she usually has to relieve one of the enders. Or, the jumper may call out the name of another jumper, to jump in as he or she jumps out.

The enders have their choice of manipulating the rope in any number of ways, and there are many versions of the game:

- High Tide—Turning the rope so that it doesn't hit the ground, then gradually raising it, making it more and more difficult for the jumper to jump. There is another game called "High Water," which requires the rope to be held above the jumper's head. The jumper must crouch down in order to jump under the rope.
- On Line—This is for multiple jumpers. They line up and must jump into the turning rope in a steady rhythm.
- Jumping Jacks—A player jumps in, jumps once, and jumps out. Then he or she jumps in, jumps twice, jumps out. The jumper keeps going, each time jumping more times in succession, until he or she misses.
- Winding the Clock—The jumper jumps in and counts to twelve, turning around on each jump.

● Baby's Cradle—The enders keep the rope swaying back and forth. The jumper(s) jumps from side to side until he or she misses. This is similar to "Snake," in which the rope is wriggled from side to side on the ground. The jumper tries to jump and avoid touching the rope, or being "bitten" by the snake.

The above is just a sampling of all the possibilities for two or more players. These can be done with two people by tying one end of the rope to a tree or pole, while an ender turns the other end.

## Double Dutch

Almost everyone remembers this two-rope game, probably the most difficult of the jumping games. The enders hold two long ropes, one in each hand, and turn both ropes inward, or outward (sometimes called "Double Irish"). One rope should be held a little higher than the other. Begin turning the lower rope, then add the higher rope while the jumper tries to jump over one, then the other, running in place quickly. It takes a lot of concentration, and much more than that if you attempt to jump to rhymes. There are many variations of Double Dutch, named after the countries in which they originated.

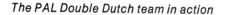

*The PAL Double Dutch team in action*

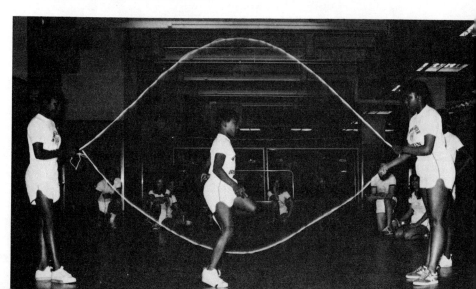

## JUMPING-ROPE RHYMES

There are thousands of jumping rhymes from all over the world and all parts of this country. Many are similar to one another, changed by regional language or slang variations. Since most of these have been handed down by word of mouth, they are considered a valuable addition to folklore literature.

Here are a few of the more universally popular rhymes. (For more, look at the Bibliography and visit your local library.)

*Strawberry shortcake*
*Cream on top,*
*Tell me the name*
*Of my sweetheart:*
*A,B,C,D,E,F,G,H,I ...*

*Teddy bear, teddy bear*
*Turn around,*
*Teddy bear, teddy bear*
*Touch the ground,*
*Teddy bear, teddy bear*
*Show your shoes,*
*Teddy bear, teddy bear*
*Go up the stairs,*
*Teddy bear, teddy bear*
*Say your prayers,*
*Teddy bear, teddy bear*
*Turn out the light,*
*Teddy bear, teddy bear*
*Spell goodnight:*
*G-O-O-D-N-I-G-H-T*

*Blondie and Dagwood went downtown,*
*Blondie bought an evening gown,*
*Dagwood bought a pair of shoes,*
*Cookie bought the daily news,*
*And here's what it said to do:*

*Close your eyes and count to ten*
*And if you miss, take an end.*

*I like coffee, I like tea,*
*I like the boys,*
*And the boys like me,*
*I'll tell my Pa*
*When I get home*
*The boys won't leave*
*The girls alone.*

*Mary [name of jumper] drinks lemonade,*
*Mary drinks beer,*
*Mary drinks other things*
*That make her feel queer.*
*"Oops," said the lemonade,*
*"Oops," said the beer,*
*"Oops," said the other things*
*That made her feel queer.*

*Oh, life is merry,*
*Life is fun,*
*That's what I tell everyone.*
*But if they don't agree with me,*
*I hope they'll be stung by a big, fat bee.*

*Cross the river, cross the sea,*
*Johnny broke a bottle*
*And blamed it on me.*
*I told Ma, Ma told Pa,*
*And Johnny got a whipping,*
*Ha! Ha! Ha!*
*How many lickings did he get?*
*1,2,3,4,5,6,7,8 . . .*

*Down in the meadow where the green grass grows,*
*Sat little* _____
*As pretty as a rose.*
*She sang, she sang, she sang so sweet,*
*Then along came* _____
*And kissed her on the cheek!*
*How many kisses did she get?*
*1,2,3,4,5,6,7,8 . . .*

*Indiana Banana*
*Played the piano,*
*But all she knew was the* Star-Spangled Banner.
*She wiggles, she wiggles,*
*She does the split,*
*But when she misses, she misses like* this.

# Chapter 5

## *The Jump-into-Super-Shape Diet*

I happened upon this wonder-working diet by accident. It has been tremendously successful for me and many of my students, and I am pleased to have the opportunity to share it with you. Let me tell you how I discovered this palate-pleasing shortcut to becoming thin.

The five-day Health and Diet Expo at the New York Coliseum in New York City was attracting thousands of people per day, and I was on an impossible schedule of twenty performances daily! Busy as I was, I couldn't help noticing that one display booth was always surrounded by a large crowd. During a break, I wandered over to see what was happening there. The center of attraction was raw food. "So, what's different here?" I thought to myself. Then I looked closely at the beautifully colored array of food and my mouth started to water. I picked a salad topped with a pretty red dressing and vegetable juice made fresh for me at the booth. I gulped down my purchase and ran to do yet another show.

Five days went by quickly. I had no time to run out and buy cooked meals. But the raw food display was near me, with its delicious salads and refreshing juices. Whenever I felt hungry, I trotted over and ate.

Now, even though I had been a professional athlete for years and worked out hours each day, I always had a tough time controling my weight. (My raging sweet tooth might have had something to do with that.) I fought the battle of the bulge at every turn. I had tried every fad diet that came out, always looking for the miracle that would leave me slim. Nothing really worked, and it looked like my fate was to enjoy and then starve.

By the third day at the coliseum, I realized I was feeling terrific! Could it be my imagination, or was I slimming down? I had come to enjoy the delicious raw foods and juices at the show. If anything, I was overindulging. How could I be getting slimmer? I weighed myself and, sure enough, I was three pounds lighter. Joy of joys, what had I discovered? *Nothing* was the answer. This was too simple to be a discovery.

I decided to investigate this phenomenon further. I made it my business to meet the man who was feeding thousands of New Yorkers each day with home-grown raw foods brought fresh from his country farm.

Viktoras Kulvinskas, author of *Survival into the 21st Century* and *Love Your Body* (see Bibliography), turned out to be my mysterious food benefactor. I listened to his lectures, read his books packed with nutritional information, and decided to go whole hog into a raw food regime. That was definitely the best decision I have ever made.

Gone were the hours of food preparation, gone were a lot of expenses. And best of all, gone were the extra pounds I had been fighting for years. I had plenty of energy and never felt heavy with food, even though I was eating as much as I wanted and my skin was glowing with health!

Satisfied with my controlled weight, I stayed on raw foods and kept my diet to myself until the members of one very large jump-rope class cornered me after a workout. This particular group contained a lot of overweight people. "Help us— you stay so trim." I just knew they'd never try it, but I took the time to tell them about my raw foods and some of the fabulous-tasting recipes I had come across. Then I forgot about it.

The next week I was almost assaulted by the enthusiasm of my already thinner students. "It works"—"I'm not hungry"— "My skin cleared up"—"I have so much energy"—these were the remarks my excited students threw at me.

Fascinated, I decided to investigate more thoroughly. I had two karate students, beautiful young women, who were both carrying a few extra pounds. They constantly dieted and gained. They hated the vicious circle, but their modeling careers demanded they stay lean. I approached them with my idea and they agreed immediately to try the diet under my watchful eye.

I monitored their diet and exercise program for fifteen days. They spent weekends with me and I prepared all their food.

The results astounded me. They both lost almost a pound a day until they reached what must have been a natural weight for their bodies. Then the weight loss stopped and they maintained a steady weight on the same diet!

Both beauties were glowing. Neither looked drawn from weight loss; both had excellent skin tone and felt marvelous.

Now, really involved, I started to research the effects of raw food on the human body and came up with some fascinating facts.

• *The aging process is much faster with cooked foods!* Nobel prize winner Dr. James Sumner (see Bibliography) tells us that the middle-aged feeling is due to the diminishing of our enzymes as we get older. We are alive today only because we contain thousands of different kinds of enzymes that regulate the life process.[1] *Only* raw foods contain health-giving, rejuvenating enzymes. Cooking, pasteurizing, smoking, pickling, and any other interference in nature's processes will denature (deprive of their natural character) enzymes, thus preventing the nutrients in food from being readily available.[2]

• *Cooked foods produce diseases!* Common cooked foods produce leukocytosis. *Leukocytosis* is the name that medical

[1] D. M. Locke, *Enzymes—The Agents of Life*
[2] A. Tannenbaum, "Nutrition and Cancer" in *Physiopathology in Cancer*

pathologists give to an excessive number of white corpuscles in the blood. The white corpuscles are the defense organisms of the blood that prevent infection and intoxication of the blood. The body's delicate balance is thrown off as cooked foods cause an increase in the white corpuscles.[3]

Many doctors and nutritionists believe that cancer and arthritis are caused by, and flourish on, cooked and refined foods. Dr. Ann Wigmore of the Hippocrates Health Institute in Boston stated, "The most thrilling experience I can recall was to see cancer cells taken from a human body thrive on cooked food but unable to survive on the same food when it was uncooked."[4]

• *Cooked food has lost more than 85 percent of its nutrient value! Vitamins are lost in the cooking process.* Here is a list of nutritional casualties that take place when you cook your food: thiamine loss in cooking is 25–45 percent and can go as high as 96.4 percent; riboflavin loss, 40–45 percent; biotin becomes generally unstable and can lose 72 percent of its value; ascorbic acid loss, 70–80 percent; vitamin A loss, 10–30 percent; vitamin E loss, 50 percent.[5] According to the U.S. Department of Agriculture, preparation and cooking can cause the loss of 45 to 55 percent of the B complex fraction in certain foods and can destroy all lecithin![6]

• *Protein is lost through cooking!* There are many experiments on the destruction of protein by heat. The U.S. Department of Agriculture sponsored one such study, which reported that the average temperature in home cooking "caused a very marked decrease (4-fold to 30-fold) in the soluble protein nitrogen of steak."[7]

[3]F. J. Ingelfinger, *For Want of an Enzyme*
[4]Ann Wigmore, *Be Your Own Doctor*
[5]B. W. Beadle, Cheldelin, Elvehjem, Farrer, Fritz, Harris, *see* Bibliog.
[6]U.S. Dept. of Agriculture, *Information Bulletin 112*
[7]F. T. Beard, *Effects of Aging and Cooking on the Distribution of Certain Amino Acids and Nitrogen in Beef Muscle*

• *Raw vegetable juices are healing.*[8] My research on vegetable juices resulted in my purchasing a vegetable juicer. It is definitely the best investment I ever made, and I can't figure out how I got along without one before.

• *Carrot juice* is used to treat all sorts of illnesses successfully. The optic system is particularly nourished by carrot juice.

• *Celery juice* contains an exceptionally high percentage of vital organic sodium. It is one of the most valuable juices for people who have used concentrated sugars and starches consistently all their lives.

• *Cucumber juice* is the best natural diuretic known. It is also known for its helpful promotion of hair growth due to its high silicon and sulphur content.

• *Dandelion juice* is exceedingly high in potassium, calcium, and sodium. It is our richest source of magnesium and iron. Magnesium is essential for preventing softness of the bones.

• *Green Pepper juice* is abundant with silicon, greatly needed by the nails, hair, tear ducts, and sebaceous glands. When properly combined with carrot juice, it is noted for quickly clearing up skin blemishes.

• *Parsley juice* (parsley is actually an herb) has properties essential to oxygen metabolism which help maintain normal action of adrenal and thyroid glands. Raw parsley is so potent that *it must never be taken alone in quantities of more than one ounce at a time.*

I suggest that you read up on vegetable juices and find out which delicious combinations are best suited for you and your needs. The vegetable juice books listed in the Bibliography will give you formulas for combining juices.

If you don't have a vegetable juicer, use fruit juices. Don't drink juices out of cans! Your juices must be made and used fresh if you are to reap benefits.

---

[8]N. W. Walker, *Raw Vegetable Juices*

- *Raw foods fight arthritis.*[9]
- *Raw foods are good for your heart! Raw foods are good for your intestines!* Raw fruits and vegetables will provide you with all the fiber and bulk you need to keep your intestines in tip-top shape. They are natural laxatives. There is no cholesterol in fruits and vegetables. High cholesterol levels can lead to heart disease (see chapter six). In fact, in Great Britain the insurance companies give better policy rates to vegetarians.
- *Raw foods contribute to a longer life!* The peoples noted for longevity—Georgians, Ecuadorians, Hunzas, and so on—exist mainly on raw foods. The small amounts of protein in their diets come from sprouts; their only meat and dairy comes from goats.
- *Sprouts are a complete protein![10] Sprouts are high in vitamins.* All the nutrients needed for healthy growth and reproduction can be obtained from sprouts. The abundant amount of chlorophyll found in sprouts (especially alfalfa sprouts) helps to minimize the destructive effect of pollution. Wheat sprouts are one of the best examples of vitamin content. In three days of sprouting, their weight doubles and they become sweet. In four days of sprouting, the vitamin E content increases 300 percent. Some of the components of the vitamin B complex show an increase of from 20 percent to 600 percent!
- *Fresh fruits and fruit juices cleanse the human system.* Viktoras Kulvinskas says: "On a diet high in fruit, urine, saliva and skin secretions become alkaline, and also have the taste and fragrance of the fruit eaten. Such a body is a delight to companions and to God."
- *Natural sugars in vegetables and fruits take the place of "junk" foods and lessen the craving for sweets.* One friend who was a sugar addict was helped by drinking raw vegetable juices

---

[9]Viktoras Kulvinskas, *Survival into the 21st Century.* Ann Wigmore, *Be Your Own Doctor.* Max Warmbrand N.D., D.C., D.O. *Overcoming Arthritis and Other Rheumatic Diseases. How Thousands of My Arthritis Patients Regained Their Health*

[10]Kulvinskas, *Survival into the 21st Century*

whenever the craving hit. After a while, and plenty of raw juices, his desire for refined sugars completely left. So, if this is your problem, don't try to fight it. Just drink plenty of vegetable juices.[11] Eat lots of fresh fruits and vegetables and Mother Nature will fix you right up!

After researching modern-day nutritional advice and raw food facts, I turned to the ancient scriptures. Over and over again, I found beautiful references to living foods: "I do say to you: Kill neither men, nor beast, nor yet the food which goes into your mouth. For if you eat living food the same will quicken you, but if you kill your food, the dead food will kill you also. For life comes only from life and death always comes from death" (Jesus, *Essene Gospel of Peace*).

I found many references to sprouted foods: "Moisten your wheat, that the Angel of Water may enter it. Then set it in the air, that the Angel of Air may embrace it. And leave it from morning to evening beneath the sun, that the Angel of Sunshine may descend upon it" (Jesus, *Essene Gospel of John*).

Lastly, I queried all the doctors and therapists whose advice we heeded in matters of the heart (see chapter Six). All agreed that a raw food diet was a healthy one.

So, jumpers, if you'd like to drop some pounds, or just generally get yourself into supershape, here's the diet for you. Now, you may ask, "Why diet if jumping rope burns lots of calories?"

Exercise will burn calories but not as many as we'd like to think: it takes twenty-six minutes of jogging to burn off one ice-cream soda, and six minutes of bicycling to atone for one little chocolate chip cookie. An hour of rope skipping will burn about 300 calories.[12] So, you can lose weight just by jumping rope, but it will take time, and the weight loss will be gradual.

If you have been existing on a diet of refined and cooked foods, you may experience some discomfort when switching to all raw foods. Consult your doctor or nutritionist. Perhaps you

[11]Walker, *Raw Vegetable Juices*. L. Newman, *Make Your Juicer Your Drugstore*
[12]Frank Konishi, *Exercise Equivalents for Weight Watchers*

will want to ease into a total raw food regime. And read! The Bibliography in this book lists some wonderful sources for informing yourself. Go to your local health food store—most of them have informative reading material on raw foods.

Exercise decreases the appetite. Therefore, if you are dieting, try to jump rope before each meal. Even if it's just for a couple of minutes, the brief workout will decrease your hunger!

Be adventuresome with the raw fish recipes—they are delicious. And since all call for marinating the fish in lemon, you will notice that the lemon "cooks" the fish a bit. The fish will turn color as though it were exposed to flame! I have served guests raw fish dishes and have waited until the compliments came before telling them their food was cooked by nature.

Try growing your own sprouts. It's so easy, and if there are children in your home, it's a great way to teach them about nutrition. Here's a simple way to grow sprouts (my favorite are alfalfa). Even if you are a city-dweller, you can have a window garden that will produce delicious whole meals.

## GENERAL SPROUTING METHOD

*Buy a large mason jar.* Remove the inner disk from the lid and replace it with copper screen, plastic window mesh, nylon, or cheese cloth—whatever's easiest and handiest for you. Just a piece of cheesecloth, held on with a rubber band, is fine.

*Wash your seeds thoroughly and soak overnight,* at least two parts water to one part seeds. Use water of a tepid temperature. The smaller the seed, the less soaking time needed. Alfalfa will do with only three hours but won't be harmed by up to fifteen. Larger seeds, such as chickpea, soy, and mung, may be soaked up to twenty hours.

In the morning, after the initial soaking, *turn your jar upside down* and *pour off the water* (the mesh will allow the water to go, the seeds to remain). *Rinse the seeds and pour off the water again.* Now *place the jar in a dark place, upside down and slightly tipped,* so that air can enter. *Rinse twice a day. On the third day, place your sprouts in the window.* The sun will turn

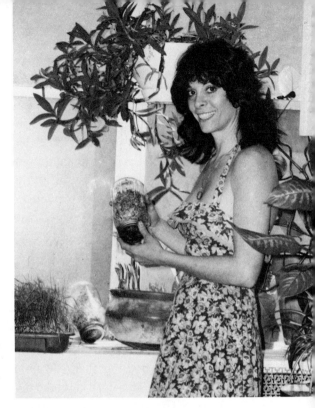

*Sidney Filson grows
wheat grass
sprouts and
comfrey in
her apartment
window garden*

them green with healthy chlorophyll. Make sure you wash your sprouts twice a day and always have the jar tipped so air enters. The sprouts are ready to eat after one day's exposure to the sun.

You might also try growing wheatgrass. Read about its wonderful powers![13]

Experiment with different kinds of seeds and find your favorite.

One of the great advantages of living on raw foods is that there are no forbidden foods. You may have anything you want, as long as it's raw! This is certainly different from most weight-loss diets where certain fruits are allowed but others are taboo because of high calorie counts. I've included a chart of fruits and vegetables with calorie counts for your own information (see pages 92–95). But don't let former calorie rules interfere with your enjoyment of this diet. Just enjoy your favorites from nature's harvest and watch your body's beautiful response. And don't forget to note the large decrease in your food bills.

[13]Kulvinskas, *Survival into the 21st Century*

Many of the following recipes have been contributed by my friends and students. If you have any terrific, delicious raw food favorites, please send them to me so that I can pass them on.

Remember, don't add anything to this diet even if you think what you're adding might be all right. I have had people fail to lose weight and come to me with complaints that this raw food regimen doesn't work. When I carefully checked their intake I found lots of mistakes.

• *Don't drink milk! Don't eat cheeses!* Consumption of dairy products is a common mistake, one that will throw your diet way off. Cow's milk is the most mucus-forming food used by human beings.[14] Cow's milk is loaded with casein—300 percent more than is contained in human milk. (Casein, by the way, is a milk by-product used as one of the most tenacious glues for cementing wood together.) Milk tends to form a large curd in the stomach. This curd can take up to forty-eight hours to eliminate.[15] Humans are not set up to absorb the protein in cow's milk—it is for calves![16] Even if it were possible to absorb protein from cow's milk, pasteurization would kill it anyway.[17]

Goat's milk is good for humans. It is compatible with human digestion from infancy to old age, as long as it is not heated! Since raw goat's milk is not that easy to come by, we are going to get all the nutrients we need out of juices. So, don't drink milk or eat dairy products while you are on this diet!

Let's get down to delicious enjoyment of a whole new way of eating. I'll give you seven afternoon and evening meals. The morning meal is not necessary—if eaten, it should be light, perhaps just juice.

Since this diet goes along with a hearty program of rope jumping, *it is necessary for you to replace all water-soluble*

[14]Kulvinskas, *Survival into the 21st Century*
[15]Walker, *Raw Vegetable Juices*
[16]H. Bieler, *Food Is Your Best Medicine*
[17]J. C. Annand, *Further Evidence in the Case Against Heated Milk Protein*

*vitamins.* So, for a super nutrition boost, get yourself on a *natural* high-potency, multiple-vitamin program.

## MORNINGS

"My fruit is better than gold, yea, than fine gold" (Proverbs 8:19).

Actually, you're better off skipping this meal altogether and giving your body at least a sixteen-hour fast from food every day. But, if you must eat, have a juicy fruit or a glass of fruit juice. *Only eat one kind of fruit at a time in the morning!* You may mix your fruit juices, but not the whole fruits. Remember, eat only because you are hungry, not out of habit!

Make sure you jump rope before breakfast!

## FRUIT TIPS

Sadly, most of the fruit available today is sprayed with pesticides. Wash your fruit very carefully, then set it in the sunshine. This will aerate your fruit and help to dissipate chemical sprays. If you have some wheatgrass, add it to the water when you wash your fruit. It is the best chemical-fighter available.

*Citrus fruits* are wonderful when in a fully ripened state. Oranges that are underripe or overripe can cause an overacid condition which could give you a sour stomach and a headache. This holds true for tomatoes and pineapples also.

When you buy oranges, check the stems. If they are orange, you know the fruit has been colored.

*Bananas* are best if you buy them green and let them ripen at home. Many dealers ripen their bananas with ethylene gas. You will know this has been done if the fruit turns evenly yellow in less than twenty-four hours. Bananas ripened naturally take four to twelve days.

*Mango* should be yellow in color before eaten.

*Papaya* will be bright yellow when ripe. Green, or underripe, papaya is known as a great digestive aid.

*Pineapple* must be purchased very ripe and heavy with juice. An unripe pineapple is high in acid content and can damage your teeth and create sores in your mouth. In the fully ripened state, the leaves can be pulled out without resistance.

*Melon* holds the most perfect nature-distilled water. It is sweet and alkaline. Always buy whole melons. When melons are open, they absorb toxic materials. A wonderfully wide variety of melons is available in all seasons. *Eat only one type of melon at a time!*

As a general rule, when combining fruit (but not at breakfast), combine according to type of seed—stone fruit (nectarine, apricot, cherry, peach), citrus, core fruit (apple, pear), and so forth. Actually, it would be better for you to eat as much as you want of one fruit at a sitting (you may make an entire meal of fruit) than to mix a lot of different kinds. This is called "mono eating" and is nature's way.

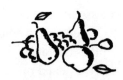

## MAIN MEAL DISHES

It is actually best to take your heaviest meal in the afternoon. This rarely fits into family plans, but try not to eat your largest meal too late in the evening. There are times when you may feel that a glass of wine is called for. If you must drink wine, stick to light white wine. Alcohol is bad for you, so try to avoid it whenever possible.

Scandinavians, Latin Americans, Polynesians, and Orientals have long known the delights of raw fish and shellfish. These dishes are now becoming generally popular. Select your fish carefully from a fish market, or catch it yourself. The eyes of the fish you select should be bright and protuberant, never dull! Flesh should be stiff, not limp. The fish should smell fresh, not "fishy." Shellfish should have tightly closed shells and feel heavy.

### Cerviche (serves two)

I first ate this delicious dish in an Argentinian restaurant in Paris. Only when I requested the recipe for this spicy delight did I become aware that it contained raw fish!

    1 medium fillet of local fish (bluefish is my favorite; any
      tasty fish will do)
    2 medium tomatoes
    1 onion (red or white)
    3 small chili peppers
    1 green pepper
    1 teaspoon tabasco sauce
    2 lemons

Remove all skin from the fish and marinate the fish in lemon juice. Fifteen minutes is enough; overnight, covered in the icebox, is terrific! You will notice the fish turning color from the lemon. That is normal—almost a "cooking" process. Cut all the other ingredients into bite-size pieces. Cut the marinated fish into bite-size pieces. Combine.

### Sashimi (serves two)

Living in the Orient taught me to enjoy raw fish dishes. This is one of my favorites.

    1 pound raw tuna, or any tasty fish
    1 lemon
    1 package dried seaweed (Nori)
    fresh ginger
    hot mustard—Japanese Wasabi paste (green horseradish)
      is best
    soy sauce

Cut the tuna into strips (no problem, as the fish is very tender). Squeeze lemon over the fish. Peel the fresh ginger and cut it into thin slices. Serve on a wooden tray.

Once at the dinner table, you may make a kind of "sandwich" out of the fish by placing a slice of tuna in a piece of the seaweed and then adding a piece of ginger and a bit of the hot mustard. Pick up this little roll with chopsticks or your fingers, dip it in the soy sauce, and be delighted.

When I have company, I usually prepare the little rolls in the kitchen and bring them to the table all ready to be dipped in individual dishes of soy sauce placed before each person.

### Steak Tartare (serves four)

Meat-eaters have a wide variety of dishes to serve raw. Here's the steak eater's favorite. This is a classic French dish.

2 pounds lean ground sirloin
dash cumin
dash cayenne
dash curry powder
¼ teaspoon thyme
½ teaspoon powdered mustard
dash tabasco sauce
dash Worcestershire sauce
Cognac or port, to taste
dash soy sauce
sea salt
black pepper, freshly ground

*Garnish*
4 egg yolks
2 tablespoons drained capers
4 teaspoons chopped parsley
2 tablespoons chopped onions

Combine the basic ingredients in a bowl; taste until you reach the seasoning you enjoy. Divide the mixture into four patties and make a hole in the middle of each for the egg yolk. Serve on individual plates. Garnish with capers, parsley, and chopped **onion.**

### Beef Strips in Vinaigrette (serves three or four)

This is another beef-eaters' favorite.

1 pound top-quality steak, trimmed of all fat
1 clove garlic
3 tablespoons olive oil
sea salt
black pepper, freshly ground
sauce vinaigrette

Slice steak thinly against the grain. Squeeze (or chop very finely) the garlic clove in a bowl. Add the oil and seasoning; use a good amount of black pepper. Let marinate for an hour. Make a sauce vinaigrette by using one tablespoon Dijon mustard as a substitute for the garlic called for. When ready to serve, put the steak in the sauce and garnish with parsley and whole capers.

### Minced Lamb (serves four)

The idea of eating raw lamb may seem strange, but raw lamb is no more exotic than steak tartare and is very popular in the Middle East. The lamb must be very fresh, devoid of fat, and ground fresh for you.

1 cup crushed raw wheat germ
¾ pound lean lamb, finely ground
½ teaspoon prepared Dijon mustard
ground nutmeg to taste
dash allspice
dash cayenne
1 teaspoon fresh mint or basil, finely chopped
sea salt
black pepper, freshly ground
1 small onion, finely chopped
½–⅔ cup olive oil
chopped fresh parsley

Soak wheat germ in cold water for ten minutes. Drain in a colander lined with cloth. Wrap cloth around wheat germ and squeeze dry. Using a large bowl, combine wheat germ, lamb, and spices. Knead until well mixed and smooth. Add seasoning to taste. Divide into four portions and make a hollow in the center of each. Fill each opening with oil, then garnish with the chopped onions and parsley.

### Breast of Chicken (serves four)

This is a popular Oriental dish. The breast can be made juicier and more tasty if it is boned and then pounded with a knife before you cut it up. Never use frozen chicken for eating raw. Remember, most supermarket chicken has been frozen, so try your local farmer and hope he's feeding his birds plain old healthy corn.

4 chicken breasts
sea salt

*Garnish*
2 cucumbers
soy sauce for dip
Wasabi paste (green horseradish), or any very hot mustard

Wash and dry the chicken breasts, then pound them. Bring a pan of water to a boil. Turn off the heat. Cut the breasts into one-inch squares. One at a time, dip the squares quickly into the hot water so that they just whiten on the outside. Place in a bowl and refrigerate. Peel and shred two cucumbers. Put them in a bowl of ice-cold water until you're ready to serve them. Place the chicken on a serving plate and garnish it with drained cucumber. Serve the horseradish and soy sauce in separate dishes.

### Lobster with Basil (serves four to six)

Raw lobster has firmer flesh and is more juicy than cooked lobster. The taste stays, instead of being boiled away.

3 lobsters
juice of 2 lemons
1 cup homemade mayonnaise
1 tablespoon finely chopped onion
3 tablespoons finely chopped celery
3 tablespoons coarsely chopped fresh basil
1 tomato
1 teaspoon chopped fresh parsley

Kill the lobster by plunging a knife into the spinal cord. Remove the meat from the shell and run under cold water until it is firm (this is a more humane way of killing the lobster than plunging it into boiling water). Place meat in a dish and squeeze lemon juice over it. Leave to marinate while you prepare the mayonnaise and seasonings. If possible, leave it for an hour. To the mayonnaise add the onion, celery, and basil. Mix well. Remove the lobster meat from the marinade and mix in the dressing. Garnish with slices of tomato and parsley.

## LUNCHES AND LIGHT MEAL DISHES

### Guacamole

1 avocado, diced
2 sweet red peppers, diced fine
2 tomatoes, diced
1 teaspoon kelp
1 lemon

Use a fork and blend avocado to a creamy consistency, leaving a few lumps for texture. Mix with lemon and seasoning to taste. Add remaining ingredients. If you like spice, add freshly minced chili pepper or oil from crushed garlic.

### Stuffed Tomatoes with Shrimp (serves four)
 1 pound shrimp, washed and shelled
 juice of two lemons
 4 large, firm tomatoes
 1 cup mayonnaise
 1 teaspoon cayenne pepper
 1 teaspoon fresh parsley, chopped
 sea salt
 black pepper, freshly ground
 2 teaspoons fresh dill, chopped

Marinate shrimp in lemon juice for three hours, until pink. Hollow out a cavity in each tomato. Salt the cavity. Remove shrimp from the marinade, add seasonings to mayonnaise, chop the shrimp coarsely, and turn in the sauce. Fill the tomatoes with this mixture, sprinkle cayenne pepper on top, and decorate with parsley.

### Eggplant and Watercress Salad (serves four)
 1 small eggplant
 sea salt
 cider vinegar
 1 bunch watercress
 1 tablespoon Spanish onion, chopped
 1 tomato, sliced
 ¼ pound black olives
 1 teaspoon fresh basil, chopped
 1 teaspoon fresh parsley, chopped
 sauce vinaigrette

Skin and chop the eggplant into small pieces. Salt well and leave for about an hour. Dry off the salt and marinate the eggplant in vinegar for about three hours. Dry and put in salad bowl. Add the watercress, onion, tomato, olives, and herbs. Mix. Prepare a sauce vinaigrette. Toss and serve.

### Mushrooms Stuffed with Green Garlic (serves four)

This dish may be prepared the day before eating, as it improves when left overnight.

    1 pound large mushrooms
    2 cloves garlic
    1 tablespoon spinach leaves
    1 tablespoon chopped parsley
    1 tablespoon watercress
    1 teaspoon chives
    1 teaspoon Dijon mustard
    2 tablespoons vinegar (apple cider)
    ½–¾ cup olive oil
    sea salt
    black pepper, freshly ground

Remove stalks from mushrooms and set aside the caps. In a bowl, squeeze garlic (or chop very fine). Chop the vegetables (you can use scissors), and add them to the garlic. Add the rest of the ingredients, check seasoning, then stuff the mixture into the mushroom caps. Place mushrooms upside down, on a plate. Refrigerate until ready to serve. The liquid in the mixture will be absorbed by the mushrooms, enhancing their flavor.

### Root Salad (serves two)

    ½ cup carrots, grated
    ½ cup red beets, grated
    ¼ cup radishes, grated or finely chopped
    1 teaspoon salad herbs
    1 teaspoon honey
    1 tablespoon horseradish

Mix all ingredients well, add olive oil and lemon juice. Serve on a bed of chopped spinach or lettuce leaves.

### Celery Nut Loaf with Sauce (serves four)
2 cups celery, grated and drained
1 cup raw almonds, ground
1 avocado, mashed
3 tablespoons onion, minced
3 tablespoons parsley, minced
½ teaspoon of sage or thyme
juice of one small lemon
2 tablespoons mayonnaise

Mix the above ingredients thoroughly in a bowl. Shape into a loaf.

*Sauce*
4 tomatoes
juice of 1 lemon
1 teaspoon honey
½ teaspoon thyme and marjoram
dash of hot chili

Put all ingredients in blender, blend well, and top the nut loaf.

### Avocado and Orange Salad (serves four)
1 cup fresh orange juice
1 teaspoon orange peel, finely grated
1 dried red chili pepper, crushed
1 teaspoon fresh ginger, grated
1 cup carrots, grated
2 avocados
3 tablespoons lemon juice
3 tablespoons olive oil
½ cup raisins, soaked in equal amount warm water
sea salt
black pepper, freshly ground

Combine the orange juice, orange peel, dried pepper. Add the ginger, seasonings, and carrots. Leave this mixture for an hour at room temperature. Meanwhile, soak the raisins. When ready to serve, peel and slice the avocados and squeeze lemon juice over them to stop them from turning brown. Add the avocados to the bowl with the oil. Add the raisins, mix, season to taste, and serve.

Now you have seven main meal ideas and seven secondary meal ideas. The variations and combinations are uncountable. I have tried to give you a bit of exotica, but a plain salad is terrific for you also! Raw soups can be exciting, too.

### Borscht[18] (serves two)
    2 cups raw beets, diced.
    1 green onion
    1 cup carrot juice or beet juice or water
    1 lemon
    ½ cup almond, sesame, or coconut butter

Liquefy ingredients in blender. Delicious as a soup or salad dressing.

### Vichyssoise Verde (serves two)
    2 cups greens, chopped
    ½ avocado
    1 cup water
    1 teaspoon kelp
    Optional, choose one: 3 mint leaves, ½ clove garlic, juice
                         of 1 lemon, 1 small onion,
                         3 scallion leaves.

[18]Kulvinskas, *Love Your Body*

Use two or more varieties of greens that are in season. Swiss chard and spinach, beet tops and celery, and lettuce and celery are tasty combinations. Pour water into your blender. Add greens slowly, a little at a time. Reduce to a fine consistency. Add more greens if sauce is very thin. Blend in one optional ingredient to taste. Blend in avocado. Makes 3 cups.

Accompany your meals with salads of all varieties. All the vegetables you have been accustomed to cooking will taste wonderful raw. You'll really taste them for the first time. Personally, I was very surprised to find that corn and cauliflower are delicious raw. Combine as many vegetables as you desire in salads—be adventuresome. Use olive oil and apple cider vinegar combined with spices for dressings.

Be sure to combine sprouts for the most delicious of all salads! Alfalfa, mung, soy, and other sprouts taste wonderful together and are fine for main meal courses also.

Dessert time is always a delight. When you're on a raw food diet, you have a never-ending amount of possibilities. Here are a few of my favorites:

### Raw Applesauce (can be used to accompany main meal also)

4 apples, medium size (use juicy apples)
apple cider
juice of one-half lemon
dash nutmeg
dash powdered cinnamon
sea salt (to taste)

Peel and core the apples. Cut coarse slices and put them in the blender. Add a little cider and blend. Add the lemon juice and seasonings and blend, adding cider until you have reached a consistency that seems right to you.

## Cantaloupe Delight

1 cantaloupe per person
port wine
seedless grapes or strawberries

Open the cantaloupe by slicing off a bit of the top. Scoop out seeds, fill cavity with grapes or strawberries. Fill with port wine and refrigerate. This is a great party dessert!

## Cardamom Honey Dressing (delicious with all raw fruits)

½ pint clear honey
2 tablespoons lemon juice
1 teaspoon cardamom seed, cracked

Beat the honey with an electric mixer until it is pale and creamy. Gradually beat in the lemon juice and the cardamom seed. Pour over your favorite fruit.

Your vegetable juices are of major importance to this diet and will sometimes replace meals. Drink your juice before the meal, even though it is part of the meal. Here are some wonderfully healthy combinations for you.

*Drink at least two pints of juices per day.* The more vegetable juices you drink, the better you will feel on this super-shape-up program. Remember, you're jumping rope and should be losing plenty of fluid through perspiration. These wonderful juices will replace vitamins lost, add the ones you have been lacking all along, and decrease your appetite. (They decreased mine.) A wonderful benefit, unless your experience is different from the other jumpers who tried the diet, is a marked improvement in complexion.

The following juice combinations total one pint each, in proper proportions:

| | | |
|---|---|---|
| Carrot | 7 oz | |
| Apple | 6 oz | Reputed to aid the spleen, this formula |
| Beet | 3 oz | certainly aids the taste buds! |
| Carrot | 8 oz | |
| Beet | 3 oz | This taste delight benefits the kidneys and |
| Coconut | 5 oz | liver. |
| Carrot | 8 oz | A nectarlike, soothing drink for a sore |
| Unripe Papaya | 8 oz | stomach. Ulcers are treated with both these juices. |
| Carrot | 10 oz | Chock full of vitamins A and E. |
| Spinach | 6 oz | This is a strong drink; its healing properties are very well known—everything from tooth decay to varicose veins is fought with this vitamin-rich preparation! |

Here are some eight-ounce formulas. Remember, you can't store juices! Prepare, then drink them immediately. If they must be stored, make sure it's in glass and that no air gets to them. Even in a container, juice will lose its vitamins in three hours!

| | | |
|---|---|---|
| Carrot | 8 oz | A must for a vitamin-starved or sick body. Great for children, as a replacement for milk. This is a sweet juice. |
| Cucumber | 4 oz | This will help rid you of excess water. |
| Green Pepper | 4 oz | Your hair and nails will also benefit. |
| Carrot | 4 oz | Good for your eyes! An athletes' favorite. |
| Celery | 4 oz | Delicious way to replace sodium lost through exercise! |
| Grapefruit | 8 oz | Full of organic salicylic acid to fight arthritis. Its function within your body is to dissolve inorganic, encrusted calcium. |

Before you start combining juices on your own, do some reading on the subject. If you have an ailment you'd like to fight with nature's help, read up on the subject.[19]

[19]Walker, *Raw Vegetable Juices*

Greens of some varieties can be too potent in large amounts. Beet juice should be taken in careful amounts (not more than a wineglass each day).

It is interesting to note that you do not have to worry about insecticides sprayed on vegetables when you juice them. All the books I've read on the subject agree that the sprays remain in the fiber of the vegetable, which is discarded by the machine, leaving a pure juice for you to drink.

Also interesting is the fact that some vegetables contain vitamins that are only released when juiced and could never be obtained by chewing. The carrot is one of these wonder healers whose juice can only be released by juicing, not chewing!

When you drink vegetable and fruit juices, they do not have to pass through the many hours your digestive system takes to get vitamins into your bloodstream. Instead, they pass through your stomach lining and go directly into your bloodstream in concentrated vitamin form. It's like going to the doctor and getting a shot of medicine in your vein.[20]

This diet gives you more freedom of choice among foods than any other. Make sure you use the juices to good advantage. A day spent on just juices and fruit is a partial fast that will leave your hunger satisfied, your body weight lowered, and your head feeling clear.

Please eat sprouts every day! Please jump rope before each meal!

Between-meal snacks are not good on any diet. But if you must snack, make sure it's a vegetable and dip. (Cauliflower and broccoli are good companions to a tasty dip.)

You don't have to plan ahead on this Jump-into-Super-Shape Raw Food Diet. Just wander into any vegetable and fruit store and pick out what appeals to you that day. Anything in the store is all right, as long as it's raw.

Try to keep your meat eating to a minimum. I know it's hard

---

[20]Laura Newman, *Make Your Juicer Your Drugstore*

# RAW FOODS: PROTEIN, CALORIE, AND VITAMIN CONTENT

| Food | Quantity | Protein (grams) | Calories | Vitamins[21] |
|---|---|---|---|---|
| FRUITS (fresh, uncooked) | | | | |
| Apple, unpeeled | 1 medium | .3 | 80 | A,B,C |
| Apricot, whole | 3 small | 1.1 | 55 | A*,B,C |
| Banana | 1 medium | 1.3 | 101 | A,B,C |
| Blackberries, hulled | ½ cup | .9 | 42 | A,B,C |
| Blueberries | ½ cup | .5 | 45 | A,B,C |
| Cantaloupe, whole | 1 medium melon | 2.7 | 115 | A*,B,C* |
| Cherries | ½ cup | .8 | 41 | A,B,C |
| Fig, fresh | 1 small | .5 | 30 | A,B,C |
| Grapes, seedless | 20 grapes | .5 | 54 | B,C |
| Grapefruit, pink/red | ½ medium | .6 | 46 | B,C* |
| Mango, whole | 1 medium | .9 | 88 | A*,B,C* |
| Nectarine, whole | 1 medium | .7 | 73 | A*,C |
| Orange, whole | 1 medium | 1.6 | 77 | A*,B,C* |
| Papaya, fresh, cubed | ½ cup | 1.1 | 71 | A**,B,C |
| Peach, whole | 1 medium | .6 | 38 | B,C |
| Pear, whole | 1 medium | 1.2 | 101 | A*,B*,C |
| Pineapple, fresh, diced | ½ cup | .3 | 41 | A,B,C* |
| Plum, whole | 1 medium | .3 | 27 | A,B,C |
| Raspberries, fresh | ½ cup | .9 | 41 | A,B,C* |
| Strawberries, hulled | 1 cup | 1.0 | 53 | C* |
| Tangerine, whole | 1 medium | 1.7 | 39 | A,B,C |
| Watermelon, diced | 1 cup | .8 | 42 | B,C |

| Food | Quantity | Protein (grams) | Calories | Vitamins[21] |
|---|---|---|---|---|
| VEGETABLES (fresh, uncooked) | | | | |
| Artichoke, Jerusalem | 4 oz | 2.6 | 75 | B,C* |
| Asparagus, whole spears | 1 lb. | 6.4 | 66 | A*,B*,C* |
| Avocado, peeled, pitted | ½ medium | 2.4 | 185 | A,B,C |
| Beans, Green, 2" pieces | ½ cup | 1.0 | 17 | A*,B,C |
| Bean Sprouts: mung | ½ cup | 1.7 | 16 | A*,B,C |
| soybean | ½ cup | 3.3 | 25 | A*,B,C |
| Beets, diced | ½ cup | 1.1 | 29 | A,B,C* |
| Broccoli | ½ cup | 2.4 | 20 | A*,B,C |
| | 8 sprouts | 6.5 | 56 | A*,B,C |
| Cabbage, red or white | 1 cup shredded | 1.2 | 22 | B,C* |
| Carrot | 1" x 6", medium | 6 | 21 | A*,B,C |
| Cauliflower, flowerets | ½ cup | 1.4 | 14 | A,B,C* |
| Celeriac Root, pared | 4 oz | 2.0 | 45 | |
| Celery | 1 large stalk | .4 | 7 | A*,B,C |
| Chard, trimmed | 4 oz | 2.7 | 28 | A**,B,C |
| Chives, cut | 1 oz | .5 | 8 | C |
| Chicory Greens, trimmed | 4 oz | 2.0 | 23 | A*,B,C |
| Corn, raw kernels | 4 oz | 4.0 | 109 | A*,B,C |
| Cucumber, peeled | 6 slices | .3 | 7 | A,B*,C |
| Dandelion Greens | 4 oz | 3.0 | 51 | A**,B,C |
| Endive, Belgian, trimmed | ½ cup | .3 | 4 | A*,B,C |
| Escarole, in pieces | 1 cup | 1.2 | 14 | A*,B,C |
| Kohlrabi, diced | 1 cup | 2.8 | 40 | B,C* |

| Food | Quantity | Protein (grams) | Calories | Vitamins[21] |
|---|---|---|---|---|
| Lettuce, Iceberg, chopped | 1 cup | .5 | 8 | A*,B,C |
| Romaine, shredded | ½ cup | .3 | 4 | A**,B,C |
| Mushrooms, sliced | ½ cup | .9 | 10 | B* |
| Onion, chopped | 1 tablespoon | .1 | 4 | B,C |
| Onion, Green (Scallion) | 3 small | .3 | 11 | A*,C |
| Parsley, chopped | 1 tablespoon | .1 | 2 | A*,C* |
| Peas, Green, shelled | ½ cup | 4.3 | 58 | |
| Peapods, Chinese (Snow) | 4 oz | 3.3 | 49 | |
| Pepper, Green, seeded | 1 medium | .7 | 13 | A*,B,C |
| Potato, slices, raw | 1 cup | 3.1 | 113 | A,B,C* |
| Radishes, whole | 1 cup | 1.3 | 22 | B,C* |
| Rutabaga, diced | ½ cup | .8 | 32 | B,C* |
| Spinach, whole leaves | 1 cup | 1.1 | 9 | A**,B*,C** |
| Squash, Summer | ½ cup | 1.0 | 15 | A*,B,C |
| Tomato, whole | 1 medium | 1.6 | 33 | A*,B,C |
| Watercress | ½ cup | .4 | 3 | A*,B,C |

MISCELLANEOUS

FISH (fresh, raw)

| Food | Quantity | Protein (grams) | Calories | Vitamins[21] |
|---|---|---|---|---|
| Clams | 4 medium | 10.7 | 65 | |
| Flounder, fillet | 4 oz | 18.9 | 90 | |
| Oysters | 12-19 medium | 20.2 | 158 | |

| Food | Quantity | Protein (grams) | Calories | Vitamins[21] |
|---|---|---|---|---|
| Salmon, raw | 4 oz | 25.5 | 246 | |
|   smoked | 4 oz | 21.3 | 221 | |
| Scallops | 4 oz | 17.4 | 92 | |
| Shrimps | 4 oz | 20.5 | 103 | |
| Sole, fillet | 4 oz | 18.9 | 90 | |
| | | | | |
| SEEDS | | | | |
| Pumpkin, hulled | 1 oz | 8.2 | 157 | |
| Sesame, hulled | 1 oz | 5.2 | 165 | |
| Soybean, roasted | 1 oz | 10.8 | 145 | |
| Sunflower, hulled | 1 oz | 6.8 | 159 | |
| | | | | |
| TOFU (SOYBEAN CURD) | 4.2 oz cake | 9.4 | 86 | |

[21] Asterisk denotes high levels of vitamin indicated.

if you're used to eating meat every day, but as long as you're changing shape, why not let your insides relax for one week?

Your whole family will benefit from this diet, even if they are not jumping rope with you. They will enjoy the different way of eating for one week also. Children grow like flowers on this diet!

Happy jumping into super shape! I know you're going to look great!

# Chapter 6

## Jumping for Your Heart and Health

Jumping rope is considered an aerobic exercise. You may already know what makes some exercises aerobic and how aerobic training benefits the overall health of your heart, lungs, and circulatory system. But if you're still mystified about what this all means and *why* aerobic exercise promotes cardiovascular fitness, let's get down to some basic explanations.

### WHAT IS AEROBIC EXERCISE?

*Aerobic* sounds like mumbo-jumbo from the new vocabulary of the Space Age, but it simply means *with oxygen*. So, if you are aerobically fit, you will be able to exercise at a good fast pace and yet maintain sustained, relaxed breathing. Aerobics have been popularized by Dr. Kenneth Cooper (see Bibliography). His physical fitness programs have been adopted by millions of people, as well as by the U.S. and Canadian armed forces.

The term *aerobic* refers to an exercise activity's ability to stimulate one's use of oxygen, thus enabling the body to produce the energy needed to carry out muscular work. So, aerobic

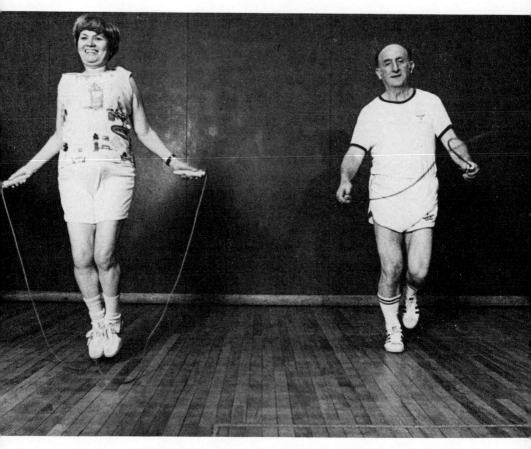

*Sarese and Joseph—good sports with healthy hearts*

power, or endurance, is directly related to your capacity for taking in oxygen.

Dr. Richard Stein, Director of the Cardiac Exercise Laboratory at the State University of New York's Downtown Medical Center, explains it this way: "When you get into exercise training, a lot of things happen. There's an improvement in cardiac efficiency—your heart has to do less work to meet your body's needs at each stage of working intensity."

"For example," Stein continues, "you might try running up a flight of stairs and then take your pulse. Say the count is 120. If you spent thirty minutes running up and down stairs, three times a week, at the end of that week your pulse would be lower, say 100."

"Assuming that your body weight remains the same, your muscles would need the same amount of blood as they did the first time you climbed the stairs. Your heart would have to pump the same amount of blood. But now it will be able to pump *more* blood with each beat, and therefore will have to beat less often. By beating less often, the heart itself requires less oxygen, and will work efficiently on less oxygen at each given load of exercise." So, aerobic conditioning is cardiovascular conditioning.

Only certain exercises (e.g., jumping rope, jogging, swimming, stair climbing, bench-stepping, cycling) have been proven to effectively develop the desired cardiovascular endurance. These exercises require the continuous rhythmic tensing and relaxing of the muscles of the legs, trunk, and to a lesser degree, the arms. When these exercises are sustained at a peak level for ten to twenty minutes, this stimulates one's blood flow and promotes cardiovascular endurance. The exerciser also experiences an increase in body temperature, heart and breathing rates, and sweating.

With aerobic conditioning, you will be able to do long stretches of work because your body is receiving and utilizing enough oxygen to break down the waste products that are produced by exercise.

## WHAT ARE ANAEROBIC AND INTERMITTENT EXERCISES?

There are high-intensity exercises of short duration (e.g., the 100-yard sprint) that are termed *anaerobic,* meaning *without oxygen.* Since these exercises cannot be sustained for a long period of time, they do not improve one's cardiovascular fitness.

Likewise, *intermittent* exercises—isometrics, weightlifting, calisthenics, ballet exercises, yoga, and many sports (golf, bowling, skiing, volleyball, tennis, squash,[1] etc.)—will tone your muscles and improve your athletic ability. But they will not increase your oxygen intake. Only aerobic exercise will promote "good wind."

## WHAT IS "CARDIOVASCULAR FITNESS"?

*Cardiovascular* pertains to the integrated performance of the heart and blood vessels. *Cardiorespiratory* refers to the action between the heart and the lungs. Cardiovascular fitness —total physical fitness—is the condition which exists when a person is able to exercise strenuously for long periods of time, *without fatigue.*

In other words, when you are in good shape you will have the stamina to work long and hard without straining your heart, lungs, and circulatory system. As Dr. Stein says, "You will be able to pump more blood with less effort."

## WHAT ARE OTHER BENEFITS OF A GOOD EXERCISE TRAINING PROGRAM?

You will be less fatigued and will have more energy. Studies have shown that people who exercise regularly also reduce their use of tranquilizers and sleeping pills.

"Once you start to do one good thing for yourself, like exer-

---

[1]Sports such as tennis and squash can be considered aerobic only in singles, with the play strenuously continuous for thirty minutes or more, three times a week.

cise," Dr. Stein points out, "you begin to do other good things for yourself, like diet and health care. People become a little more ritualistic about taking care of themselves when they exercise. They begin watching what they eat, their weight begins to drop, and they feel good."

Many psychiatrists, in fact, put their patients on a physical exercise regimen, because they feel that exercise can become a "positive addiction" in a world full of many negative influences. The body and the mind work together. Therefore, something that's good for the body, like exercise, will also be good for the mind.

## HOW DOES THE HEART BENEFIT FROM EXERCISE?

An exercise fitness program—such as rope jumping—that enhances your cardiovascular endurance will decrease your chances of ever having a heart attack, or having another if you've already suffered one. And if you should ever have a heart attack, chances are that it will be milder if you are in good physical condition.

We all know that when we exercise we look and feel better. We have more energy. Now, research into "exercise physiology" is proving that exercise, especially in this age of American leisure, may help us live longer. Even cardiac patients, once confined to life in an easy chair, are strengthening their hearts and blood vessels with exercise. This has been made possible by the "stress test," a means of scientifically measuring the amount of exercise a person can undertake without danger.

[2]In scientific studies (such as ones conducted with Harvard graduates and with San Francisco Bay dock workers) it has been proven that people who exercise tend to have fewer heart attacks than people who do not. At a meeting of the American Heart Association (Miami Beach, November 1977), Dr. Ralph Paffenbarger, Jr., presented the findings of a ten-year study (conducted at the Stanford University School of Medicine) indicating that exercise has been shown to reduce the risk of heart disease by about 60 percent, a very significant amount.

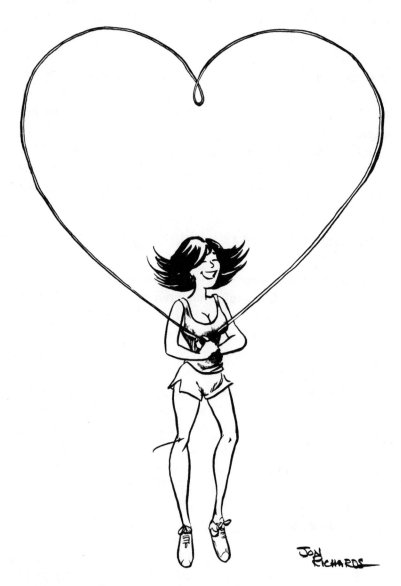

*Be good to your heart—start jumping!*

## WHAT CAN EXERCISE DO FOR THE CARDIAC PATIENT?

Dr. Stein states: "Noncontrolled studies indicate that you'll live longer if you exercise after a heart attack than if you don't exercise. But we have no real evidence that exercise does anything for the disease itself. We know that, in studies with animals, exercise has stopped atherosclerosis and has increased the growth of collateral blood vessels around obstructed vessels. But it has never been proved with humans. I can't actually say that you'll live longer after a heart attack if you exercise, but you will improve the *way* in which you live after a heart attack if you exercise."

Basically, aerobic exercises, such as jumping rope, train your heart to pump more blood with each beat. This is desirable for cardiac patients because the heart will become a "better muscle," according to Dr. Stein.

Frequently, patients who have undergone exercise programs no longer need drugs for chest pain. Dr. Stein reports that such patients often have fewer palpitations, less pain, less shortness of breath, and less stress during sexual activity. "In fact," he says, "there is an increase in the frequency of sexual activity and gratification after a heart attack if you exercise."

## EXACTLY WHY IS ROPE JUMPING CONSIDERED AN AEROBIC EXERCISE?

Garry Neupert, of New York's Cardio-Metric Institute, explains it this way: "To develop a person's cardiovascular endurance, an exercise must involve at least 45 percent of one's total body muscle mass. Jumping rope meets this criteria because it uses almost all of the muscles from the waist down, to varying degrees, as well as the muscles of the arms and upper body."

"Jumping rope," continues Neupert, "also meets the three other conditions necessary for cardiovascular enhancement: intensity, duration and frequency."

In order to understand more fully, let's elaborate:

• Intensity—one must exercise at the appropriate intensity (between 60 and 85 percent of a persons's predicted maximal heart rate) to sufficiently stress or overload one's cardiovascular system and promote endurance.

• Duration—the exercise must be performed for a minimum of ten minutes at this 60- to 85-percent intensity range. (Obviously, the more work you do over a longer period of time, the quicker your endurance will be improved.)

• Frequency—the exercise must be performed at least three times a week, on alternate days.

## MUST AEROBIC EXERCISE BE PERFORMED NONSTOP, OR CAN YOU REST?

The Cardio-Metrics Institute emphasizes that there is no significant difference whether the required threshold time is performed with frequent rest pauses ("interval, or intermittent training") or with no rest pauses ("continuous training").

## WHAT IS INTERVAL TRAINING?

Interval training breaks your exercise period into shorter "sets" of work and rest (stretch). "If you exercise for three minutes, and then rest (walk around or stretch) for two minutes," says Dr. Stein, "and do this four times in a row, you will have twenty minutes of excellent conditioning."

"The rest intervals seem to add into the training time. You exhaust yourself, then regenerate—one, then the other—and this process stimulates muscles to build more each time. The rest period also gives you time to check your pulse rate."

Neupert, at Cardio-Metrics, recommends interval training for the first couple of months if a person:

• has a very low exercise capacity, or poor muscular development;

• has not exercised regularly within the past ten or more years;

• is forty years or older and hasn't been checked out by a stress test. (The same recommendation applies if a person is overweight, a heavy smoker, or has a family history of heart disease or high blood pressure.)

## IS THERE A DANGER OF TOO MUCH EXERCISE, TOO FAST?

Of course. As with everything, you shouldn't overdo. Do not take up jumping rope—or any strenuous exercise regime—without a checkup, and, if possible, a stress test.

Take it easy when you exercise in very hot weather, especially if the humidity is high. While you are exercising, be on the lookout for any indications that you are overdoing it: headache, chest pains, dizziness, nausea, heart palpitations, pale or clammy skin, muscle cramps, pounding of the heart after you finish. Be in tune with your body and heed its warning signs. Read—and become familiar with—the chart of warning signals on pages 106–107.

## WHAT IS A STRESS TEST?

A stress test, also called an "exercise tolerance test," is a safety check procedure. Simply, an electrocardiogram is taken and a person's body reactions are monitored while the heart is under stress from exercise on a treadmill or stationary bicycle. The test takes from forty-five minutes to an hour.

Afterwards, a personalized exercise regimen is prescribed, based on the results of the test and the person's own particular exercise preferences. Then the person is taught how to monitor his or her own pulse and to keep track of heart-rate ranges. People who have had heart attacks can be given an exact prescription as to the amount of exercise they can perform safely, without limiting exercise entirely.

## WHO SHOULD HAVE A STRESS TEST?

Ideally, everyone over the age of forty should have a stress test. Most definitely, anyone who has had a heart attack or experienced symptoms of chest pain should have one. Also, if you have been previously sedentary or have a strong family

# OVEREXERCISE:
# WARNING SIGNALS AND WHAT TO DO
# ABOUT THEM[3]

| | SYMPTOM | CAUSE | REMEDY |
|---|---|---|---|
| **STOP** — **SEE A PHYSICIAN BEFORE RESUMING** | 1 Abnormal heart action; e.g.<br>—pulse becoming irregular<br>—fluttering, jumping or palpitations in chest or throat<br>—sudden burst of rapid heartbeats<br>—sudden very slow pulse when a moment before it had been on target.<br>(Immediate or delayed) | Extrasystoles (extra heart beats), dropped heart beats, or disorders of cardiac rhythm. This may or may not be dangerous and should be checked out by physician. | Consult physician before resuming exercise program. He may provide medication to temporarily eliminate the problem and allow you to safely resume your exercise program, or you may have a completely harmless kind of cardiac rhythm disorder. |
| | 2 Pain or pressure in the center of the chest or the arm or throat precipitated by exercise or following exercise.<br>(Immediate or delayed) | Possible heart pain. | Consult physician before resuming exercise program. |
| | 3 Dizziness, lightheadedness, sudden incoordination, confusion, cold sweat, glassy stare, pallor, blueness or fainting.<br>(Immediate) | Insufficient blood to the brain. | Do not try to cool down. Stop exercise and lie down with feet elevated, or put head down between legs until symptoms pass. Later consult physician before next exercise session. |
| **REMEDIES WHICH MAY BE SELF-ADMINISTERED** | 4 Persistent rapid heart action near the target level even 5-10 minutes after the exercise was stopped.<br>(Immediate) | Exercise is probably too vigorous. | Keep heart rate at lower end of target zone or below. Increase the vigor of exercise more slowly. If these measures do not control the excessively high recovery heart rate, consult physician. |
| | 5 Flare up of arthritic condition or gout which usually occurs in hips, knees, ankles, or big toe (weight bearing joints).<br>(Immediate or delayed) | Trauma to joints which are particularly vulnerable. | If you are familiar with how to quiet these flare-ups of your old joint condition, use your usual remedies. Rest up and do not resume your exercise program until the condition subsides. Then resume the exercise at a lower level with protective footwear on softer surfaces, or select other exercises which will put less strain on the impaired joints; e.g. swimming will be better for people with arthritis of the hips since it can be done mostly with the arms. If this is new arthritis, or if there is no response to usual remedies, see physician. |

| SYMPTOM | CAUSE | REMEDY |
|---|---|---|
| 6 Nausea or vomiting after exercise. (Immediate) | Not enough oxygen to the intestine. You are either exercising too vigorously or cooling down too quickly. | Exercise less vigorously and be sure to take a more gradual and longer cool-down. |
| 7 Extreme breathlessness lasting more than 10 minutes after stopping exercise. (Immediate) | Exercise is too taxing to your cardiovascular system or lungs. | Stay at the lower end of your target range. If symptoms persist, do even less than target level. Be sure that while you are exercising you are not too breathless to talk to a companion. |
| 8 Prolonged fatigue even 24 hours later. (Delayed) | Exercise is too vigorous. | Stay at lower end of target range or below. Increase level more gradually. |
| 9 Shin splints (pain on the front or sides of lower leg). (Delayed) | Inflammation of the fascia connecting the leg bones, or muscle tears where muscles of the lower leg connect to the bones. | Use shoes with thicker soles. Work out on turf which is easier on your legs. |
| 10 Insomnia which was not present prior to the exercise program. (Delayed) | Exercise is too vigorous. | Stay at lower end of target range or below. Increase intensity of exercise gradually. |
| 11 Pain in the calf muscles which occurs on heavy exercise but not at rest. (Immediate) | May be due to muscle cramps due to lack of use of these muscles, or exercising on hard surfaces. | Use shoes with thicker soles, cool down adequately. Muscle cramps should clear up after a few sessions. |
| | May also be due to poor circulation to the legs (call claudication). | If "muscle cramps" do not subside, circulation is probably faulty. Try another type of exercise; e.g. bicycling instead of jogging in order to use different muscles. |
| 12 Side stitch (sticking under the ribs while exercising). (Immediate) | Diaphragm spasm. The diaphragm is the large muscle which separates the chest from the abdomen. | Lean forward while sitting, attempting to push the abdominal organs up against the diaphragm. |
| 13 Charley horse or muscle-bound feeling. (Immediate or delayed) | Muscles are deconditioned and unaccustomed to exercise. | Take hot bath and usual headache remedy. Next exercise should be less strenuous. |

[3]This chart reprinted by permission from *Beyond Diet . . . Exercise Your Way to Fitness and Heart Health* by Lenore R. Zohman, M.D. Published by CPC International Inc. Copyright © 1974. (See Bibliography.)

history of heart disease or high blood pressure, you should undergo a stress test.

Dr. Stein specifies: "Anyone who has one of the risk factors associated with heart disease (heavy smoking, high cholesterol, obesity, a high-stress job) probably should have a 'maximum' stress test done, in a medical center rather than a doctor's office."

### IS A MEDICAL CHECKUP ALSO NECESSARY?

Yes, have a medical checkup even if you plan to have a stress test. Before beginning any program of strenuous exercise like jumping rope, you should have your doctor's approval, especially if you have been inactive or are overweight. Make sure this checkup includes: a resting electrocardiogram, a blood analysis (for cholesterol and triglycerides), and an examination of the cardiovascular system, blood pressure, muscles, and joints.

### HOW HIGH SHOULD YOUR HEART RATE BE WHEN EXERCISING?

This depends on your age and health. "The maximal heart rate or oxygen intake," explains Neupert, "is determined individually through stress-testing. But if this isn't possible, a person can arrive at a fairly good estimate of his threshold level by using the established pulse rate values for his age range."

Dr. Stein elaborates, "If you can train and sustain a target heart rate that is about 75 percent (or between 60 and 85 percent) of your maximum heart rate for a period of about twenty to thirty minutes, you would have the ideal training response for a minimum amount of effort."

As you exercise, your heart rate goes up until it reaches a steady state, pumping blood to your muscles. As you become fit, your heart will have to work less to pump the same amount of blood into your muscles.

To pick your target rate, look at the chart for the average target range for your age. Then, immediately after you have exercised, take your pulse and refer to the chart to see if you're on target. If your pulse/heart beats per minute are *over* target,

## MAXIMAL ATTAINABLE HEART RATE
## AND TARGET ZONE[4]

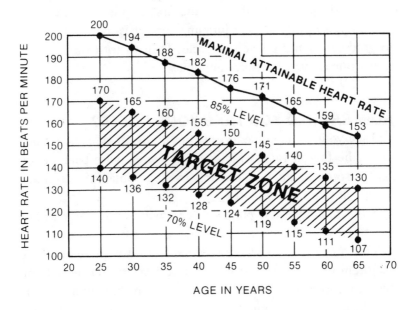

This figure shows that as we grow older, the highest heart rate which can be reached during all-out effort falls. These numerical values are "average" values for age. Note that one-third of the population may differ from these values. It is quite possible that a normal fifty-year-old man may have a maximum heart rate of 195 or that a thirty-year-old man might have a maximum of only 168. The same limitations apply to the 70 percent and 85 percent of maximum lines.

[4]This chart reprinted by permission from *Beyond Diet . . . Exercise Your Way to Fitness and Heart Health* by Lenore R. Zohman, M.D. Published by CPC International Inc. Copyright © 1974. (See Bibliography.)

cut down either the intensity or the duration of the exercise: jump less vigorously and less high; put a minute of gentle skipping into the middle of your workout. If your pulse rate is *under* what it should be on the target range, it means you're not working hard enough.

Dr. Stein points out that for the first couple of weeks in a new exercise program like jumping rope it is more important to gradually build up your muscles than to try to match the target rate of heartbeats per minute.

## HOW SHOULD YOU TAKE YOUR PULSE?

Take your pulse immediately after you stop an exercise, because the fall-off rate is rapid. Locate your pulse beat, count for ten seconds, and then multiply by six to obtain the accurate heartbeat rate for a minute.

You can count your pulse beats (which are the same as the heart rate) by placing your hand over your heart, or over any of the other locations where you can feel a full pulse beat: on the thumb side of the wrist, the carotid artery[5] on the side of the neck, inside the bend of the elbow, on the temples, or in the groin. (Practice finding your pulse when you are resting, so you'll know where it is.) It is easier to find the pulse after exercising because the beat is more apparent.

The fall-off rate of heartbeats per minute is so fast that it is necessary to locate your pulse and take it the instant you have finished exercising. However, if you continue to feel a rapid pulse five minutes after exercising, it's an indication that you should have a stress test. The same goes for a prolonged state of exhaustion after exercising. The stress test will tell you whether this is a danger or caused by the fact that you are simply out of shape from being inactive.

---

[5]To locate the carotid artery, find the bend of your jawbone with your finger and move it down about half an inch. Press extremely lightly here—never press both sides at the same time. Stop if you become dizzy.

## WILL EXERCISE REDUCE CHOLESTEROL AND TRIGLYCERIDES IN THE BLOOD?

There is a reduction of triglycerides as long as you continue to exercise, but if you stop your exercise program the triglyceride count goes back up. There is no evidence that exercise lowers cholesterol. Cholesterol can be controlled only by a diet which is low in saturated fats and red meat.

## WHAT HAPPENS WHEN YOU STOP AN EXERCISE PROGRAM?

There is no indication that it's bad for you to exercise for a while and then stop. But you will lose all the benefits you've worked so hard to gain. The detraining effect, or fall-off of fitness, occurs rapidly—almost 60 percent in three weeks. If you hurt yourself and stop exercising for six weeks, you will be back at the starting gate when you begin training again.

## CAN ELDERLY PEOPLE JUMP ROPE?

Jumping rope is generally considered too exhausting for anyone who has been previous sedentary. But an older person who has been relatively active and whose stress test results allow, can jump rope. In fact, it's an ideal exercise because it can be done at home, indoors.

## HOW NECESSARY IS THE WARM-UP BEFORE EXERCISING?

Warm-up is important. If your muscles are warm when you begin your exercise, you will perform better. You will be able to do more with less fatigue, and there will be a decrease of stress on your heart if you warm up.

In the case of jumping rope, the jumping *is* the warm-up, especially if you start off slowly with the rest stop. Other warm-up exercises include running in place, high stepping in place, and walking briskly.

## WILL THE EXERTION OF JUMPING ROPE CAUSE SOME WOMEN TO URINATE INVOLUNTARILY?

Dr. Herbert Schwartz, New York City obstetrician and gynecologist, says, "Jumping rope will not cause this condition, but if it already exists the condition will react to jumping rope."

The condition occurs most often, but not exclusively, in women who have had multiple childbirths. It is due to a dropped bladder. If you find that this happens to you when you begin jumping rope, consult your doctor.

## IS IT TOO LATE TO START TRAINING TO IMPROVE YOUR HEART'S FITNESS?

No! The consensus is that people are trainable at any age, from twenty to seventy—even if they have been leading the typical sedentary American lifestyle.

So, get your jump rope out and go to it! It's never too late to get in shape.

# Chapter 7

# *The Social Jumper*

If you are lonely and would like to find a friend, take your jump rope somewhere, anywhere! If you jump rope near other human beings, you are bound to make new friends. It's a good bet that someone you attract while jumping will say, "Hey, I used to be pretty good at that. May I try your rope?" The full bloom of nostalgia has taken over. Hardly anyone can resist the urge to flash back to childhood.

It's funny. People who normally would never speak to strangers—let alone ask to borrow form them—will zero right in on your rope. Go ahead—let them have a crack at it. Now that you know how to jump, you'll get a kick out of watching others try. (Just keep your chuckles to yourself when they trip, which they will.) The typical rope borrower usually returns the rope quickly, with an embarrassed, "I'll have to get back into that one of these days." Of course, other people watching the scene will have elevated you to expert status by now. They will be anxious to discuss your skill, make friends, or have you teach them how to jump.

The word *social* means "marked by friendly companionship," which could also define jumping rope. So, if you'd like to measure your wealth in friends and haven't found your people yet, get your treasure chest ready. Jump ropes attract kindred souls like friendly magnets!

> "Your friend is your needs answered."
> Kahlil Gibran, *The Prophet*

My mother had moved to the sunshine state of Florida, but ill health prevented her from getting outside. She had been there for six months when I arrived for a visit. In all that time, she hadn't met a soul or ventured to the wonderful beach nearby.

My visit perked her up and she was feeling better, so off we went to the beach. Of course, I had my trusty rope with me, as well as a small cassette player and tapes of my favorite jumping music. As my mother watched, I jumped rope.

At this point let me warn potential beach jumpers: showing off by the waterside can be tricky. The sand does *not* support your feet like a hard surface, and you jump yourself into a hole. I wish someone had warned me!

While I struggled to remain above sea level, my mother proudly extolled my virtues as a rope jumper to the gathering crowd. My problems with the sand steadily increased, and my calves began to burn like crazy. As I gamely tried not to let Mom down, I was overjoyed to hear the familiar: "Can I try?" I handed over my rope with no further ado and sat down to watch the borrower sink into the sand. I turned to my mother to let her in on the joke, but I couldn't get her attention: she was too busy exchanging phone numbers and talking local politics. My social rope had done it again!

> "And in the sweetness of friendship
> let there be laughter and sharing of pleasures."
> Kahlil Gibran, *The Prophet*

A national magazine did an article about my rope jumping which brought in thousands of letters and calls. Swamped with work at the time, I couldn't deal with most of the requests for

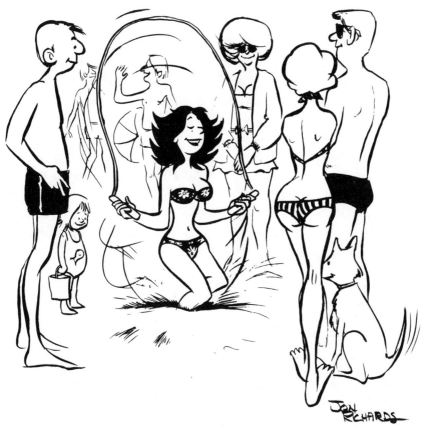

*The hazard of beach jumping*

advice and lessons, but one call really aroused my curiosity. It was from two middle-aged women, roommates; one was sixty, the other sixty-five. I arranged to give them a semiprivate lesson.

My two students arrived on time, with the right equipment and exactly the right attitude. We had a wonderful class. Both women gave me their full concentration, and we were able to go beyond my usual agenda for a first class. In a healthy sweat after the good workout, we all sat down to chat.

The older woman, of European background, was retired and now worked for an agency which employs senior citizens part-time. Her roommate, a black American, worked full-time at an advertising agency but was retiring soon. The women had decided to live together to ease their financial burdens, and the arrangement was working out wonderfully. Spurring each other on, they had switched to natural foods and eliminated all chemical intake. They sported a few extra pounds but assured me that they were already dieting. Only two things were lacking: "A good exercise program and a social life." At least I had solved their workout worries.

I prescribed a maintenance program, gave them a list of music to jump by, and wished them well. I had really enjoyed the lesson. They were superior women, both witty and good natured. And they were enthralled with their newly learned skill as they affectionately kissed me goodbye. I made them promise to call if they had problems or forgot anything technical.

*Teddy and Barbara on a jump rope date*

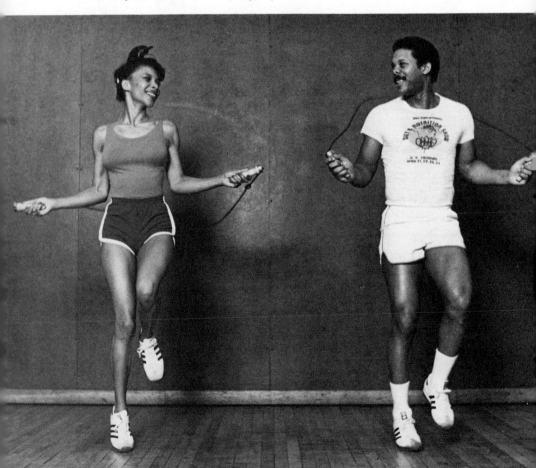

A few days later, the women called, in a dilemma. It seems that they had been diligently jumping in their apartment every day, until their cranky downstairs neighbor complained about the noise. They were only jumping lightly, the building they lived in was not well-constructed. The neighbor's complaints put a stop to the women's jumping.

"What shall we do?" they lamented.

Luckily, it was springtime. I found out that in front of their building there was a cemented area with a few benches. The tenants, mostly senior citizens, went there to take a bit of sun and have some neighborly gossip. I advised the women to take their ropes outside, along with a tape player for their music.

At first, they wouldn't consider it. They would be "too embarrassed" to jump in public. But then again, they really liked to jump. Finally, they got up their courage and went out with their ropes. They found a secluded corner away from the other tenants, who they were sure would object to their disco music and ropes.

As it turned out, they attracted so much friendly curiosity and admiration that they were urged to hold an outdoor class for the whole building. The cranky downstairs neighbor ended up apologizing for her attitude and asked to join the class. By the time cold weather came around, most of the building's residents were turned on to rope jumping. The tenants got together and persuaded the management to turn a basement storage room into a workout area and social club.

Time and time again, I've seen lonely people turn into social butterflies after learning how to jump rope.

My friend Marty had another kind of problem. He was tongue-tied when it came to first meetings with the opposite sex. He had a great job, was very good looking, but just couldn't get started on a conversation with a woman. All of his vacations were spent traveling around the world. Every time he'd go off on a new jaunt, he hoped to meet an interesting woman. When he returned home he always used the same excuse: he couldn't speak foreign languages. At least that's what he told me.

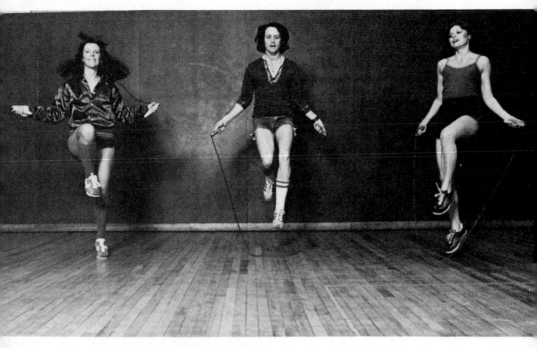

*Jonathan makes friends with Beverly and Claudia,*
*thanks to the "social rope"*

Marty finally solved his problem with a jump rope. We made
a wager and he promised to carry out his part. So, in the middle
of health- and beauty-conscious Scandinavia, surrounded by the
tall, blond beauties he was longing to date, he took his jump rope
to the city square. In front of the fountain where everyone
gathered to hang out, he turned on his cassette player loaded
with American disco music and jumped rope for twenty minutes, nonstop.

Needless to say, I won my bet. Marty created a small sensa-
tion. The language barrier was broken by sound and sight, and
he was invited to a party that evening. And, by the way, the
snapshot I later received of him, arm in arm with a glorious,
golden-haired young woman, strongly indicated native companionship!

Marty paid off the bet. Every time I look up a word in the
deluxe dictionary that he sent to my house, I flash back to this
story.

And let there be no purpose in friendship
save the deepening of the spirit."
Kahlil Gibran, *The Prophet*

Friendship seems to come easier in a small town. Most people in small towns have known each other since childhood. New families moving in get the "Welcome Wagon" treatment and neighbors generally tend to be helpful.

Making friends in a big city can be difficult, even dangerous. Singles bars are filled with searchers on an endless treadmill. They bask in a euphoria created by alcohol, and friendships formed this way last about as long as the effects of the liquor.

I live in a huge apartment building in New York City and have had lots of opportunities to observe my single neighbors' plights. The roof of our building is large, and when the weather gets warm, tenants go there to lie in the sun. It's both funny and sad, because it's obvious that a lot of those people would like to meet each other. There they are, lying around in bathing suits next to one another, and no one has the courage to break the ice.

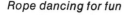

*Rope dancing for fun*

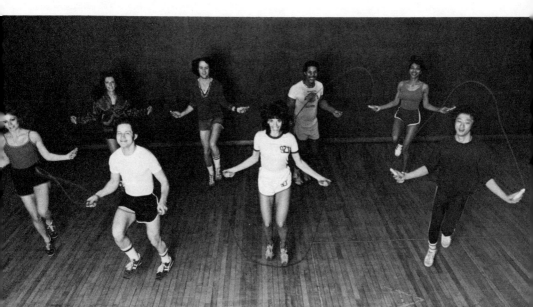

Last spring, I went up on the roof to catch a few rays but soon became bored just lying there. I needed a workout, so I ran back to my apartment and grabbed my jump rope and music.

Not wanting to disturb the twenty or so silent readers and sunbathers, I secluded myself behind a water tower. I cleared a space in the pebbled surface, put on my music, and worked out. My mind must have been far away, because I never noticed all the attention I had attracted until I finished my stint. I became the talk of the building that afternoon. I met more fellow tenants on that roof that day than in all the years I had lived in the building.

So, go ahead. Take your jump rope somewhere, anywhere. You'll find friends. But, I have one warning for you. Please heed: Showing off can be dangerous! Showing off is fun and definitely part of social jumping, but there are pitfalls to avoid. You are more likely to have an accident while showing off, because your mind is on your audience. A twisted ankle hurts and can also stop you from working out for a long time. And stepping on the rope twenty times in a row will quickly disperse your audience. So, if you're going to show off, concentrate on your perfect form and nothing else!

# Chapter 8

# Let's Go!
# Keep Going!
# There Is Nothing Else!

These wonderful words of inspiration were first boomed into my ears by the powerful voice of a famous grand master of the martial arts, Peter Urban. The phrase was meant to spur even greater efforts from his exhausted, at-the-end-of-their-rope karate students.

Already a black belt when I heard these pearls of wisdom; I had learned and practiced self-discipline. I had pushed myself hard, proven myself in the martial arts, and knew first-hand that nothing was impossible. Yet even with all this positivity, there was a little something missing. The gap was filled the moment Master Urban bellowed out the phrase that has come to mean so much to me. My back straightened, a second wind blew in from somwhere, and I felt better about everything.

Since that time, there have been many moments when I have needed that second wind: to feel better, get out of a tough situation, work harder, or overcome physical or emotional obstacles. At those times I've been able to rev up my motivation motor by saying to myself: LET'S GO! KEEP GOING! THERE *IS* NOTHING ELSE! This positive statement works for me; I hope it will do the same for you. You can try it out by applying it to the discipline of jumping rope for your scheduled fifteen-minute workout each day.

There is everything to be gained from self-discipline, including inner joy and beauty. Certainly, the day will come when, after jumping rope for ten minutes, you'll say to yourself: "I don't feel great today. I'll stop now and make it up tomorrow. What the heck—it's just five minutes!" No! Wrong! Those seemingly unimportant five minutes are extremely significant: they can change your whole lifestyle. If you make that push and jump those few minutes, you will be taking a forward step that will carry over into every aspect of your life. That lazy day will become special.

There is real satisfaction in knowing that you've helped yourself. Take a moment and reflect: how many things do you do each day that are truly beneficial for yourself? By jumping rope for fifteen minutes and not giving in to a weak moment, you've reaped an extra bonus. You're stronger now. When the next "impossible" task presents itself, when you actually come to the hurdle, you will be able to think back to the first day you pushed yourself and apply the same strategy. It *will* work.

All self-improvement books remind us that beauty is more than skin deep. Inner beauty produces a radiant glow which attracts other people, much as a flame draws a moth. Everyone wants to bask in the light and catch a bit of the magic. Self-discipline, practiced without deviation, will bring you that sought-after aura. Self-discipline, applied to rope jumping, will also give you a healthier, more beautiful body. In other words, you can't go wrong.

Of course, being human, we all tend to cut a few corners here and there. For instance, you might jump rope for ten minutes and want to take a minute break before finishing your stint. You'll rationalize by telling yourself that fifteen minutes is fifteen minutes, no matter how you put it together. Wrong! Don't take that break—you're out to build stamina. (The only exception to this applies to people who have been placed on intermittent training programs—working with frequent rest pauses —by their doctors.)

If you interrupt your workout period, you will fall into a trap. This is your opportunity to do something perfectly! The flush of accomplishment that comes with finishing a disciplined workout will be your own pat on the back. Self-satisfaction comes with that extra push. We all have a reserve tank of energy. Once you discover yours, you'll always be able to draw on that source.

In my classes, after I've taught my students the actual mechanics of rope jumping and how to build their stamina, I teach them that they can go further. Everyone can expect more of themselves than they ever realized. That's why I push my students hard.

One of my students, an older woman, tended to be a complainer. She was part of a large group learning to jump at a "Y." There was a special price for senior citizens, and this elderly jumper must have thought there was going to be an easy-going attitude to accompany the discount. During the first class, all sorts of things bothered her: her rope wasn't right, her shoes were uncomfortable, her clothes were binding, and so forth.

I ignored the complaints and hoped her attitude would improve by our next session. When I noticed her slacking off and babying herself during the second class, I put on a little pressure. I reminded her that she was there to jump, not rest. (She had remained in the rest-stretch position for over five minutes.)

Pulling herself up, she immediately defended herself: "My dear, I hope you realize you're speaking to a sixty-year-old senior citizen."

"How wonderful," I replied. "In my last jump-rope group, I had a sixty-eight-year-old woman who outjumped everyone else. I know what to expect from someone your age." (I had also reviewed her physical fitness chart, seen the results of her stress test, and knew she was fully capable of committing herself to the program.)

"But I'm tired today," she countered. "I didn't sleep well last night."

"You will tonight," I assured her.

As our bantering continued, it became important to me to

change this woman's attitude toward exercise and to stop the self-indulgence she felt entitled to because of her age. I answered each of her complaints; there were times I thought she'd throw down her rope and leave.

During the fifth class of a series of six (one per week), I witnessed a radical change in my geriatric problem-child. There she was, floating along on the rope. Good, healthy sweat was glistening on her cheeks. The music was motivating her rhythm and she had a smile on her face!

Everyone noticed the change. After class, when my changling explained her new attitude, every ear was tuned in. During the past week, she had gone out of town to visit her daughter. She hadn't seen her child for a year and was dismayed to find her overweight, out of shape, and complaining about everything. The enterprising mother taught her daughter to jump rope.

"I found myself having to prod her on," she laughed. "Me! Can you imagine?" Her visit had proved a wonderful awakening, both for her and her daughter. Having become an example of physical fitness and discipline, there was no way she could return to her prior behavior in class.

Her new attitude was terrific and still is. I see my friend whenever I teach at the "Y." She is now head of sports activities for her senior citizens group and absolutely refuses to let any of them complain that they're too old to jump rope. But when she comes out with "Let's go! Keep going! There *is* nothing else!" (which she does at the drop of a hat, in the precise, clipped tones of a drill sergeant), I have to call on my own self-discipline to keep from chuckling out loud.

## EQUIPMENT DISCIPLINE

By now, if you're serious about jumping rope, you have all of your equipment: a rope, running shoes, records, perhaps ankle weights. Since you need all these things for your workout, they should be kept together, in an easily accessible area where they won't be exposed to extreme temperatures or crowding.

It is important to always return your equipment to the same

place. Don't carry it to other parts of the house. You can miss an entire fifteen-minute workout by misplacing your gear. If you're on the way to an office in the morning, this can cause a lot of frustration.

## TIME-OF-DAY DISCIPLINE

It is better to jump in the morning. The energy that comes will sustain you throughout a hard day of work. I know that it's tempting to put off your workout until later, but it will be harder to get to after a day's work. If you've been having restless nights, then the morning workout is a must. Certainly, an evening workout is better than none. Thousands of people fill exercise classes after work, but, given the choice, you should take the early-day benefits.

## PERFECT-FORM DISCIPLINE

You have now learned the correct body form for rope jumping. You've learned where each hand belongs, where your knees should go, where your heels should not go, which parts of your body should move, and which parts should not. These things do not change.

You must always check your own form. Even if you've been jumping for a long time and are confident that you know what's correct, glance over to your hand. Make sure it's *exactly* where it belongs. (Review the illustrations in chapter three.) Perfect form will ensure perfect results—seek it.

## TEACHING-A-FRIEND DISCIPLINE

If you happen to teach a friend to jump, make sure you don't cheat him or her out of the important points you've learned. Sometimes people have a tendency to gloss over disciplines when working with friends. They feel embarrassed about demanding attention or pushing people they know well to work really hard. It is imperative, however, to teach your friends correctly. Or else don't teach them at all. Explain why, and let them read this book.

However, watch out for the tendency to go too far into discipline when teaching a friend. And make sure you know the physical condition of the person you're teaching—that is, the results of a medical checkup or stress test.

### BREAKING-A-BAD-HABIT DISCIPLINE

When you catch yourself doing something wrong repeatedly, you have a bad habit developing. Nip it in the bud! It will give you a chance to practice another wonderful form of discipline: *concentration*. The most common bad habits are using the arms too much (instead of just the wrists), touching the heels to the ground, and coming down too hard. No matter what the bad habit is, concentrate on correcting it. Put your attention on that area only. Forget everything else until you break your bad habit. If you procrastinate, you will simply be going backward. In some ways we are like computers—correct programming is necessary for desirable results.

### PAYING THE PIPER
### (WHAT TO DO THE DAY AFTER
### YOU'VE RUINED EVERYTHING!)

The day after you've missed a workout, you must *double* your workout time. Or you may break it into two workouts. You will be much less apt to break training again if you take your punishment and jump to two records instead of one: a half-hour instead of fifteen minutes. Actually, this is wonderful when it happens: paying the piper shows how fit you've become and gives you the opportunity to make everything all right again. Use the slogan at this time: LET'S GO! KEEP GOING! THERE *IS* NOTHING ELSE!

*Why* you missed your workout makes no difference (even if you don't feel it was your fault). You either jumped or you didn't, and you will have to double up the next day to atone. Besides, once you have that first half-hour jumping session under your belt, you will be very proud of yourself.

Falling off the Jump-into-Super-Shape Diet may also be paid for with double jumping sessions. *Warning:* this can become a vicious cycle. Don't get into the habit of eating now and paying tomorrow.

In general, *don't kid yourself*! I have a male friend who loves to jump rope with me. He takes his workout seriously and always comes properly equipped. I jump nonstop with him for fifteen minutes. During the workout he will come to a dead pause, wipe his brow, and say, "Whew." After the brow wipe, he takes time getting the rope back into his hands, then more time getting started again. He goes through this routine repeatedly during the workout. By the end of the record, he is fully satisfied with himself. To this day, he still refuses to believe he's not getting a good workout and cannot understand why his weight remains out of hand.

If other people want to kid themselves, that's their problem. You can tell them once that they're not working hard enough. After that, don't frustrate yourself. Concentrate on your own fitness.

## DISCIPLINE AWAY FROM HOME

No matter whether it's a business trip, a pleasure cruise, or a weekend in the country, take along your friend, the jump rope. It takes up hardly any space, weighs very little, and guarantees your returning home in better shape than ever.

Last year, I was in London on business for two weeks. I had dreaded it, knowing that there would be lots of meetings and business lunches and dinners, with very little time for keeping in shape.

My hotel room was tiny, but there was just enough space between the bed and dresser to jump rope. And so I did, faithfully, every day. I missed the music, which helps my feet fly (there was no radio), but I jumped by the clock.

My American business associates along on the trip were on the same schedule; every one of them gained a little weight each day. The raw salads I loved were not featured in the restaurants we were taken to. Most of the food swam in heavy cream sauces; sugar and salt abounded in everything.

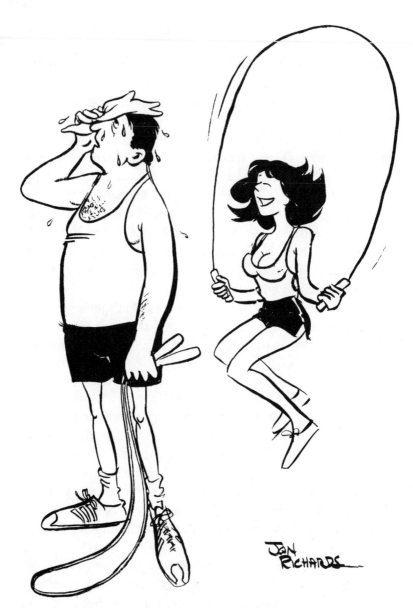

"Whew! Boy, am I tired."

Near the end of the trip, my associates began commenting that I hadn't gained weight. They were amazed when I told them about my rope jumping, and all swore to take their ropes along on their next trip.

## DISCIPLINE IS DISCIPLINE:
## NOW THAT YOU HAVE IT ...

Your discipline shouldn't only apply to jumping rope: it will work for other sports. The next new form of athletics you attempt will be easier because you know how to maintain a regimen.

Now that you've jumped yourself into shape, go ahead and learn new things. Your rope time can also be used as a fantastic warm-up for other sports or forms of movement. Many dancers jump rope before stretching their precious legs. Martial arts practitioners jump rope to warm their whole bodies before a strenuous workout. (This guards against pulled muscles.) Boxers have always known the tremendous benefits derived from the jump rope. By jumping rope; they acquire speed and timing, which are essential for the ring. Runners, joggers, cyclists, and tennis players appreciate the stamina-building qualities derived from the rope.

Good luck to you. I hope that jumping rope has enriched your life as much as it has mine and that by now you have jumped yourself into beautiful shape. Remember: LET'S GO! KEEP GOING! THERE *IS* NOTHING ELSE!

# Chapter 9

# How To Teach a Jump-Rope Class

This chapter is for anyone who wants to get together a group for a rope-jumping class, including physical education teachers. The following instructions and pointers are taken from my own experiences in teaching large classes of rope jumpers. Once you become proficient on the rope, you'll be amazed at how many people will want you to show them how to do it.

## BEFORE YOU BEGIN:

1. Have a list of necessary equipment available for all students when they sign up. If possible, list local stores that carry the right gear. (Never take a chance on people harming themselves due to inferior, inadequate equipment). The essentials are:

- The longest professional type of rope
- Running shoes, worn with socks high enough to cover calves
- For women: a good sport bra or very tight leotard, for proper support
- For men: good athletic support
- Clothing which will stretch and absorb perspiration—shorts and T-shirts, sweat suits, loose jeans, and such
- Sweat bands for forehead and wrists (optional)

2. Know the physical condition of every person in your class! Ask to have medical consent and, if possible, stress tests for pupils over forty years old. Don't fool around here: it's up to you to protect yourself and your students.

3. Prepare the musical segments of your class. Make sure the record or tape player has speakers powerful enough to be heard in the entire teaching area. Don't settle for background music; your students must be able to hear and respond to the music. If your budget allows, try to build up an adequate selection of albums. You will probably play three per session.

Select records which have a good jumping beat from beginning to end. Such albums can be hard to find, so go to your local music store and ask for assistance. A long-playing record that gives continuous jumping music will run from fifteen to eighteen minutes per side. A small 45-r.p.m. record will give you only two to three minutes per side, which means that you're much better off with albums for most of the class time. The beat doesn't always have to be fast-paced, you'll want to vary it. But waltzes by Strauss just aren't good to jump rope by.

A few 45-speed records are good to have on hand—particularly the ones on the current best-seller charts. Your younger students will relate to this music, having heard it on the radio. As your class becomes more advanced and seeks the harder, sprinting workout, you can introduce a few really fast-moving numbers.

## HOW TO TEACH A ONE-MONTH COURSE

The following is a breakdown of my rope-jumping course. I teach four classes—one session per week, sixty minutes per session.

### The First Class

1. *Line up the students and check them for equipment.* If you spot inadequate shoes, do not let the wearer jump that day. (Incredibly, some people show up in street clothes or high heels and expect to participate.)

2. While they are lined up, explain to your students that the class will be conducted with discipline. Therefore: *"No talking during class,* thank you."

3. During the lineup, give the basic rules for all jumpers:

- While jumping, breathe only through the nose.
- All steps are to be done on the balls of the feet. (Stress how lightly their feet must make contact with the ground to avoid damaging their joints. Use the phrase: "If you can *hear* your feet, you're jumping too hard!")

4. Show your students the proper way to hold the rope handle. Have everyone do it, and check each one. Point out exactly where their arms belong in relationship to their body. Explain the right angle; then show them. Stress that they are to be the center of a perfect, moving circle and that they must move only their wrists. Ask them all to try it.

5. Inform the class that there are only two things allowed during the session: jumping rope and stretching. *There is nothing else!* They may rest whenever they want, as long as they rest in the *stretch position.*

6. Demonstrate the stretch (resting) position: bend over and place your palms flat on the floor as close to your feet as possible. The jumper is to relax, breathing in through the nose and out through the mouth. Students must remain in this stretch until they feel collected and are ready to jump again.

WARNING: During this and subsequent classes, keep a sharp eye on your students (especially the older ones) for signs of overdoing; watch for dizziness, nausea, pale skin. Listen to any complaints they may have: lightheadedness, chest pains, headache, muscle cramps. Memorize the chart on the warning signals of overexercise and what to do about them (in chapter six, pages 106–107).

It is also up to you to keep your students from hurting themselves in class. Make sure that your students jump lightly, especially when they are learning new rope steps. Don't let them pound the floor as they touch down!

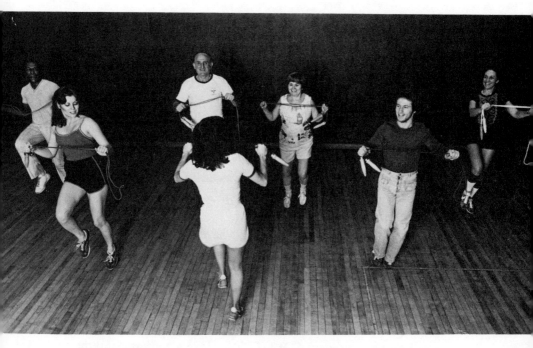

*Students should learn new steps while holding their ropes in front*

### Teaching the Steps

Now that your students know the basic rules, you're ready to go into action. It's time to get down to jumping and teaching: *The Running Step.* (See specific instructions in chapter three.) Demonstrate the step for the class, as slowly as you can. Talk while you jump. Point out how quiet your arms are, how lightly your feet touch the ground. Now, *hold your rope in front of you with both hands* and do the running step in slow motion. Stress that you are lifting your knees smartly and would like students to do the same. Ask the entire class to hold their ropes in front of them, and have them practice the running step with you.

As the class starts to move, trot up and down the lines, while still demonstrating the running step. *Always let the class see you performing the step they are supposed to be learning.* The class will have no problem doing the running step while holding the rope in front of them. After everyone is jumping lightly, tell them to try jumping *with* the rope. Now your work starts!

### Running-Step Problems—
### How to Cope with Them

1. *Bouncing between steps.* SOLUTION: Start all over. Have the student, or group of students, hold the hope in front of him or her again and do the running step slowly with you. Continue to take your class back to this procedure until they master it. Explain that by bouncing they are doing another step, which they will learn later. (Some people need to hear another step before they can grasp the running step, as the comparison helps everything come together.)

2. *Single footing*—bringing the same foot forward for each step instead of changing. SOLUTION: Go back to holding rope in front, and practice slow motion work.

3. *Running forward.* SOLUTION: Have the student pick a mark on the floor and stay on it. Tell your people to think "up," instead of "forward."

4. *Jumping too hard.* SOLUTION: Have a contest. Stop the class and jump for them, pointing out that your feet make absolutely no noise. Have the students jump one at a time as the rest of the class listens. This will make each person very conscious of jumping lightly. (This is of major importance. Jumping too hard can do a lot of damage to bodies—the joints, kidneys, small bones in the feet, and such.)

### Stretching Time

Stop the whole class from working, no matter what stage they are at. Take a refreshing stretch with them. Make sure they expel all air as they go down for their stretch. Tell them to breathe in through their nose and out through their mouth. *Make sure no one is bouncing after bending over.* Have them maintain the stretch position and totally relax as they listen to you.

### Instructor's Speech to New Rope-Jumpers

The following words should be repeated *exactly* to your students! This speech should be repeated *every time* the students stretch during the first class:

"Your calves are going to hurt tomorrow—no matter what kind of condition you are in. This is a new exercise for you. The stretching you are doing now will help. It will also be beneficial to keep your calves warm after class. Keep your high socks on. If possible, take a sauna or steam bath. Be sure to rub your calves with liniment *very hard:* try to get right down to the bone when you massage. Massage as soon after this class as possible! *Expect* your calves to hurt. You haven't been using these muscles and they are lax. Don't baby yourself when you feel the calf-ache tomorrow: practice your rope jumping just the same. Don't get mad at me—I'm warning you. Get mad at yourself for being in poor shape."

## Jumping

After stretching, everyone should be rested and ready for more jumping. Go back to the running step for about one minute. Don't worry about the people who are unable to stop bouncing. Eventually, they will.

## Stretching

Have the class go back into a stretch. *Repeat the speech about the calves.* Make sure everyone is relaxed and breathing correctly. Have the students concentrate on the long muscles in the back of the legs. Emphasize that their knees should be locked back, their legs perfectly straight. Talk to them in a low, relaxed voice. Soothe them.

## Jumping

*The Rest Step* (see specific instructions in chapter three). It's time to teach a second step, even if there are a lot of people who haven't perfected the running step. Learning the rest step will help them enormously. You'll see.

Line up the students again. Show them the rest step, very slowly. Tell the people who have been bouncing on the running step that their time has come—they can bounce! The bouncers will love this and will instantly relate to the new step. Speak in a low voice as you demonstrate the rest step. Explain that this step is for resting, that it is like a slow jogging as opposed to full-out running or sprinting. As you take the two beats on each step, explain it to the class as: jump and rest, jump and rest. The more relaxed *you* appear, the more your students will relax and actually rest on this step.

Now, have the class try the rest step. Most will master it with ease. Make a joke of it: "Everyone always gets the rest step." Go up and down the line of students. Correct each one individually, and *tell them when they are correct!* This is as important as pointing out mistakes and is a wonderful confidence-builder. Keep your eye on the upper body of each student. Make sure it remains quiet. Remind students to keep their thumbs where they should be on the rope handles.

*Don't* compromise on their form. If anyone looks tired, have them drop into a stretch. Never push anyone in the first class. Let each person work at his or her own pace.

### Stretching

Again, give your students the speech about their calves. Go over proper breathing and rope-holding rules. Relax the class.

### Jumping

Go back to the *running step*. Start them all over again with it. You will note that students who had problems with this step will be all right now that they have the rest step for comparison. Spend a minute or two reviewing the running step. Now, go to *doubles*. Before demonstrating doubles, (see chapter three for instructions), let your students know that you won't have to teach them anything. Everyone can do doubles. Just remind them to jump lightly and to remain flexible in the knees. Show them; then have them do doubles for half a minute.

### Stretching

Give the speech about calf stretching again while they are relaxing.

## Jumping

Have the whole class watch as you demonstrate jumping rope to *music*. Go from the *running step* to the *rest step* to *doubles*, moving slowly, then fast. Smile. Show them how much fun it is.

Have the entire class try dancing on the rope. While they are working, go from student to student. By now, you should have the lay of the land and know which of your charges are physically oriented to rope jumping and which are having trouble. *Divide your students into two groups.* The faster learners can jump in a group and entertain each other. Work with your people who are having a tough time of it. Be patient. They *will* get it together. Just because someone has a hard time in the beginning means very little in the grand scheme of your class. That person will often surprise you and end up out-jumping everyone else. It is *your* responsibility to whip your class into shape and to see that no one becomes discouraged. Make light of problems. Banter a bit, and try to keep the students who are having problems as relaxed as possible. Compliment them on the things they do correctly!

## Stop the Music

That's enough jumping. Actually, you have only worked your people for seven or eight full minutes on the rope. But this is as much as they can handle in the first class. Don't push them any harder than that!

## Leg Raises

Have your students lie on their backs, palms under their buttocks, chins resting on chests. (See chapter three for instructions on leg raises.) Watch everyone's breathing: make sure it's relaxed. Don't allow moaning and groaning—it takes too much energy to make all that noise. Frowns and grimaces require a lot of muscle work, so tell your students to put all their energy into their middles. Make sure heads are in the right position. (Placing the chin on the chest takes pressure off the lower spine.)

Check to see that their hands are under their buttocks. (This also takes pressure off the back and allows for concentration on the abdominal muscles.) Do not allow your students to drop their heels to the floor with a bang! Heels should not touch the floor between leg raises; they should be kept about an inch off the floor. Have your students do *ten leg raises*, while you count for them. Let them relax, breathing in through the nose, out through the mouth. *Do ten more leg raises.*

Have everyone place their hands by their sides and close their eyes. Tell them to breathe in through the nose, out through the mouth. Have them relax all the muscles they've worked so hard.

While your students are relaxed and lying down, advise them to jump a little each day, practicing what they have learned in class. *Repeat the speech about the calves.* I usually suggest that they replace the water-soluble vitamins lost through perspiration. (See the Bibliography for books on vitamins.) Then thank them and dismiss the class.

There will, of course, be after-class questions. It's always best to answer questions at this point rather than before or during the class. Overweight people will want to discuss diet. If you tell them about the Super-Shape-Up raw foods diet (see chapter five), they will tell you a better way. Most overweight people consider themselves diet experts, and it's a waste of time to try to convince them differently. For those interested, I often bring a list of books on diet and nutrition (see Bibliography) for the students to copy.

## THE SECOND CLASS

The beginning of the second class will introduce you to the crybabies in your group. Typical crybaby lines are: "I was crippled all week"; "I'm mad at you"; and "I had to go to the doctor." One particularly frustrating statement that instructors hear is: "You should have told us our calves would hurt!" (This in spite of the excessive warnings issued in the first class about calf pain.)

So, prepare to meet the onslaught. You haven't hurt them or done anything wrong. And although they may swear differently, many of these people probably neglected to take the care recommended in the first class. (I've taught a lot of senior citizens to jump, and so far not one has complained of muscle ache.)

If you are teaching your class in a new location, you might alert the management, since these crybabies just might complain and cause them to doubt your prowess as an instructor. However, the truth is that these people are out of shape. Their poor calf muscles are so neglected that they have to pay with muscle aches; there's no other way. My experience has taught me that these people have a bad exercise attitude. Of course they hurt, but so do other people who never mention it.

Tell them to *welcome* the pain—it means that their bodies are coming alive. Try to kid them out of their complaints. A good line to throw at a woman would be: "You only jumped rope for a few minutes. Imagine how you'd feel if you were drafted and thrown into basic training!"

Let your class know that their calves will never hurt that much again. They are over the hump, and jumping rope is the best thing that has ever happened to them. Tell them that *now* they can begin to work seriously at getting into shape.

### Review the First Class

Line the students up. Quickly run over the steps they have learned: the running step, the rest step, and doubles. Review each step separately, repeating the names of the steps. *Repeat the rules for breathing and stretching.*

### Music

Put on a record for *five minutes*. Let the class work on the previous steps and concentrate on going smoothly from one step into another. Right away, you will see which students did their homework. *Separate the group*, so that the people who need your help are together. For individual help, put them right back to holding the rope in front of their bodies and jumping in slow motion.

### Stretching

Have the class bend over and stretch, palms to the floor. Push them a bit further now. Their legs are warm and they can do better than they did in the first class.

### Jumping

Line the students up and demonstrate a new step: *toe taps* (see chapter three for illustration). As you show them the step, explain that it is a weight shift. They *must* stay in one spot for this step. Demonstrate slowly.

Now, with their ropes held in front of them, have the class do toe taps.

### Music

Put on a record for *five minutes*. Everyone should now jump to the music, adding the toe taps to their routine. You will have to spend the rest of the class on this step, stressing perfection of form.

### Toe-Tap Problems—How to Cope With Them

1. *Jumping too far from side to side.* SOLUTION: With rope in front, work in slow motion. Tell them that side-to-side is another step which they will learn later.

2. *Jumping, then tapping with a delayed action.* SOLUTION: As usual, repeat the slow-motion work. Stress that the jump and tap must occur at the same time.

### Stretching

Put the class into the stretch position. Talk them into complete relaxation. Make sure that their knees are locked in place and that they are breathing in through the nose and out through the mouth.

### Leg Raises

With the class on the floor in proper position, count out *ten leg raises*. Relax the class. Count out *ten more leg raises*. Then, another brief pause for relaxation.

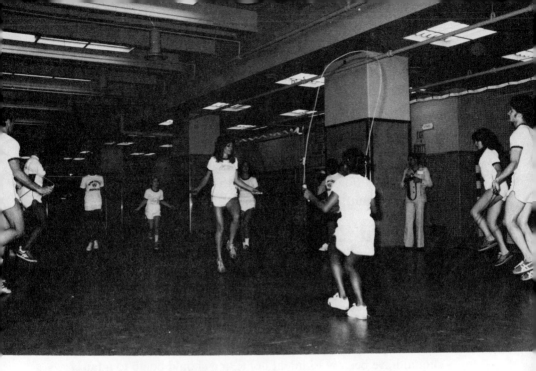

*Always let your students see you jump—*
*show them how relaxed you are*

### Stretching

Lead the class into a *floor stretch* (see chapter three for illustration) with legs open, feet flexed, and chest to the floor. Give them a good long stretch here. Go from student to student, working with this stretch.

### Music

Another *five minutes* of music. Get the class back to work, again trying to make the changes from step to step as smooth as possible.

### Stretching

Put the class into a standing stretch; then repeat the floor stretch.

### Leg Raises

Make sure each person is in the proper position. Count for them: *ten leg raises*. Relax. Now, *another ten raises*. Watch to see that legs are kept straight, with knees locked.

## Relaxation

While the class is relaxing, with eyes closed and arms by their sides, remind your students of the rules. Stress that they must take care of their calves. Make a point of telling them that they must jump at home every day, and that the next class will be a harder workout! At the end of class, answer questions.

## THE THIRD CLASS

Let your students know in the beginning that you expect more hard work in this class.

### Review Previous Classes

Put on *music for ten minutes*. Review all the steps learned so far: running, rest step, doubles, and toe taps. Your students should have been working at home and should be up to a fairly good level of stamina by now. Even though this is only your third encounter wtih them, they are three weeks into their conditioning program. Watch their form; make sure they are changing smoothly from step to step. Remind them to keep their mouths closed while jumping—*nose breathing only*. Otherwise, you'll wind up with an exhausted class. Work individually with the slower people.

### Stretching

Do both the standing stretch and the floor stretch.

### Jumping

Line the class up. Show them the next step: *the X-step—side and forward* (see chapter three for illustration). Now that the class has learned several variations, they will pick up new steps easily. Have the class practice the X-step. Work with the slower people.

### Leg Raises

Increase the count to *fifteen* per set in the third class. Remember, *you* have to teach these people to push themselves.

Fifteen leg raises. Relax. Fifteen more. There's only one class remaining, so while they relax give them a pep talk.

## Jumping

Demonstrate the next step: *side-to-side jumps* (see chapter three for illustration). Have the class practice these jumps. Have the students jump from side to side over an imaginary line. If you are working in a gym with lines actually painted on the floor, so much the better.

## Music

Put on a record for *ten minutes*. The class has a good variety of steps now. Make sure you set a good example by jumping in front, so they can see the smooth transition from step to step.

## Stretching

Do floor stretches, reaching for an optimum stretch. Extol the virtues of cleansing perspiration.

## Jumping

Demonstrate another step: the *sprinting step* (see chapter three for illustration). Have the class work at sprinting on the rope.

## Music

Put on another *ten minutes* of music. You'll have to initiate the sprinting session, as students seldom do it of their own free will. Dance in front of the class and show them all the steps you will teach them in the next, final session. This will spur them on, since everyone wants to learn the very fancy steps.

None of the steps learned in the third class involve any special problems. If you happen to encounter some, resort to your good old standby—slow-motion work.

## Stretching

Get the class into a deep floor stretch.

## Leg Raises

Count out two sets of *fifteen*, relaxing in between.

## Relaxation

As the class relaxes, still on their backs with eyes closed, give them more pep talk. Give them slogans on the importance of self-discipline. Stress the importance of practicing at home every day.

## THE FOURTH (FINAL) CLASS

Your students should feel like old pros by now. It's time to go on to bigger and better things.

## Jumping

Demonstrate *arm crosses* (see chapter three for illustration). Emphasize the even crossing of the arms and hitting the floor with the rope. Have the class try arm crosses. Expect to spend some time working on these.

Demonstrate *backward jumping* (see chapter three for illustration). Most of the steps that they have learned can be done backward.

Have the class try backward jumping. Expect the student who has been having a tough time with every other step to excel here. Some people are naturally oriented backward. Jumpers who relate to this step will be able to do all the fancy footwork while jumping backward.

*Demonstrate standing and moving figure eights* (see chapter three for illustration). Warn the class not to swing the rope wildly or they will hurt themselves (or others). Remind them to keep their elbows close to the body, for greater control. Make sure there is enough space between students.

## Jumping to Music

Put on a record for *fifteen minutes*. This is the level they are supposed to work up to and keep doing at home. Tell them so. Have them review new and old material. Keep them revved up.

It's the last class, so concentrate on their form. Be picky! Call for the sprinting step. Work with your problem-people. Remind students of the steps they are not using.

### Resting
Put them on their backs, and give them a one-minute rest.

### Leg Raises
Go into counting *twenty leg raises,* straight through.

### Jumping to Music
Divide the class into two groups. Put your stars in one group, the slower people in the other. Put on music for *fifteen minutes.* During this period, show your advanced people every step they can absorb (see chapter four). By now, some jumpers can pick up anything you show them. Since it's the last class, give them all you've got. Encourage them to invent new steps of their own. (I've had students teach me things at this point!) Work with your slower people. Remind them how much they have progressed in the past four weeks.

### Stretching
Have the class do advanced floor stretching.

### Leg Raises
Do a count of *twenty,* straight through. Then have the class relax for a full minute.

### Music
Put on a fast 45-r.p.m. record *(two to three minutes).* This is a short, fast, rhythmic jump—it calls for their very best dancing on the rope.

### Leg Raises
An extra bonus, just because it's the last class: *twenty.*

### Relaxation
While they are relaxing, go over all basic rules. Tell them

that only this last class was a truly acceptable workout. Urge them to stick to this pattern: to push themselves and not slack off. Give them the slogan: *Let's go! Keep going! There is nothing else!* They have done sixty leg raises in this class. If they are out of shape, they should do at least this many per day, although 100 would be preferable.

And, last, warn them not to become frustrated if they go into a regression period and keep tripping on the rope. This is very common. They should pay no attention and continue jumping; the problem will pass.

Thank them, and tell them to return to class whenever they need a booster shot of discipline.

# Bibliography

The following is a list of useful books and pamphlets on exercise, health, diet, and nutrition. In addition to these sources, local libraries offer myriad reference volumes, periodicals, and other resources concerning these topics.

## Exercise, Health, and Jump-Rope Rhymes

Adams, Edwin Hubbard. *Jump-Rope Rhymes.* Seattle: The Silver Quoin Press, 1947.

Ald, Roy. *Jump for Joy!* New York: Bernard Geis, 1971.

American Heart Association. *Exercise Testing and Training of Apparently Healthy Individuals: A Handbook for Physicians.* Published by American Heart Association, 7320 Greenville Avenue, Dallas, Texas 75231.

Baker, John A. *Comparison of Rope Skipping and Jogging as Methods of Improving Cardiovascular Efficiency of College Men.* Washington, D.C.: *Research Quarterly* (American Association for Health, Physical Education, and Recreation), May 1968.

Butler, Francelia, and Gail Haley. *The Skip Rope Book.* New York: The Dial Press, 1963.

Cooper, Kenneth H. *Aerobics.* New York: Bantam Books, 1972.

Cooper, Mildred, and Kenneth H. Cooper. *Aerobics for Women.* New York: Bantam Books, 1972.

Fox, Edward L., and Donald K. Matthews. *Interval Training: Conditioning for Sports and General Fitness.* Philadelphia: W. B. Saunders Company, 1974.

_____*The Physiological Basis of Physical Education and Athletics.* Philadelphia: W. B. Saunders Company, 1976.

Gray, Henry. *Gray's Anatomy*. Philadelphia: Running Press, 1973.

Halsman, Philippe. *Jump Book*. New York: Simon & Schuster, 1959.

Jessup, Claudia, and Sidney Filson. "Jump into Shape!" *Family Circle* (April 5, 1977) and "Now—An Exercise to Flatten Your Stomach in Just 7 Days," *Family Circle* (February 3, 1978).

Konishi, Frank. *Exercise Equivalents for Weight Watchers*. Carbondale, Ill.: Southern Illinois University Press, 1972.

Mitchell, Curtis. *The Perfect Exercise—The Hop, Skip and Jump Way to Health*. New York: Simon & Schuster, 1976.

Nulton, Lucy. "Jump Rope Rhymes as Folklore Literature," *Journal of American Folklore* (January—March, 1948), pp. 53–67.

Prentup, Frank B. *Skipping the Rope for Fun and Fitness*. Boulder, Col.: Pruett Publishing Company, 1963.

Rodahl, Kaare. *Be Fit for Life*. New York: Funk & Wagnalls, 1966.

*Royal Canadian Air Force SBX Plan for Physical Fitness*. Ottawa, Canada: Queen's Printer and Controller of Stationery, 1962.

Skolnik, Peter L. *Jump Rope*. New York: Workman Publishing Company, 1974.

Smith, Paul. *Rope Skipping, Rhythms, Routines, Rhymes*. Freeport, N.Y.: New York Educational Activities, Inc., 1969.

U.S. President's Council on Physical Fitness. *Adult Physical Fitness*. Washington, D.C.: Government Printing Office, 1963.

White, Paul Dudley, and Curtis Mitchell. *Fitness for the Whole Family*. New York: Doubleday, 1964.

Zohman, Lenore R. *Beyond Diet: Exercise Your Way to Fitness and Heart Health*. Englewood Cliffs, N.J.: CPC International, Inc., 1974. (Presented as a public service. Single copies *only* may be ordered from: Health Program Coordinator, Best Foods, CPC International, International Plaza, Englewood Cliffs, New Jersey 07632.)

## Diet and Nutrition

Bieler, Henry G. *Food Is Your Best Medicine*. New York: Random House, 1965.

Bircher-Benner Clinic. *Bircher-Benner Raw Food and Juices Nutrition Plan*. New York: Jove Books, 1977.

Boie, Shirley A. *Cook-Less Recipes, Raw Food Diet Plan*, and *My Adoption of a Raw Food Diet*. Los Angeles: Boie Enterprises (Box 66235, Los Angeles, California 90066).

Chase, Alice. *Nutrition for Health*. Englewood Cliffs, N.J.: Prentice-Hall, 1967.

Davis, Adelle. *Let's Eat Right to Keep Fit*. New York: Harcourt Brace Jovanovich, 1970.

_____ *Let's Get Well*. New York: Harcourt Brace Jovanovich, 1965.

_____ *Let's Have Healthy Children*. New York: Harcourt Brace Jovanovich, 1972.

Fisher, Patty, and Arnold Bender. *The Value of Foods.* New York: Oxford University Press, 1975.

Fredericks, Carlton. *The Nutrition Handbook: Your Key to Good Health.* Chatsworth, California: Major Books, 1975.

Gregory, Dick. *Dick Gregory's Natural Diet for Folks Who Eat.* New York: Harper & Row, 1973.

Hauser, Gaylord. *Look Younger, Live Longer,* New York: Farrar, Straus & Giroux, 1951.

Hodgson, Moira, *The Quick and Easy Raw Food Cookbook.* New York: Grosset & Dunlap, 1971.

Kraus, Barbara. *The Barbara Kraus Dictionary of Protein.* New York: Harper & Row, 1975.

_____ *The Dictionary of Calories and Carbohydrates.* New York: Grosset & Dunlap, 1973.

_____ *The Dictionary of Sodium, Fats and Cholesterol.* New York: Grosset & Dunlap, 1974.

Kremer, William F., and Laura Kremer. *The Doctor's Metabolic Diet.* New York: Crown Publishers, 1976.

Kulvinskas, Viktoras. *Love Your Body* and *Survival into the 21st Century.* Omangod Press, P.O. Box 255, Wethersfield, Connecticut 06109, 1975.

Lamb, Lawrence E. *Metabolics: Putting Your Food Energy to Work.* New York: Harper & Row, 1974.

_____ *Stay Youthful and Fit: A Doctor's Guide.* New York: Harper & Row, 1974.

_____ *Your Heart and How to Live with It.* New York: Viking Press, 1969.

Lappe, Frances Moore. *Diet for a Small Planet.* New York: Ballantine Books, 1971.

Locke, David M. *Enzymes—The Agents of Life.* New York: Crown, 1969.

Lust, John. *Drink Your Troubles Away.* New York: Benedict Lust Publications, 1967.

Null, Gary. *Food Combining Handbook,* and *Protein for Vegetarians.* Denver: Aurora Book Companions (Box 5852), Denver, Colorado 80217.

Null, Gary, and Steve Null. *The Complete Handbook of Nutrition.* New York: Dell Publications, 1973.

Passwater, Richard. *Supernutrition: The Megavitamin Revolution.* New York: The Dial Press, 1975.

Rodale, J. I. *The Complete Book of Vitamins* and *The Complete Book of Food and Nutrition.* Emmaus, Pa.: Rodale Press.

Sumner, J. B. *The Secret of Life—Enzymes.* Chicago: National Enzyme Co.

Tannenbaum, A. "Nutrition and Cancer" in *Physiopathology in Cancer,* Homburger, F. and Shubik, P., eds. White Plains, N.Y.: Phiebig, 1975. 2 vols.

U.S. Department of Agriculture. *Nutritive Value of Foods.* U.S. Department of Agriculture Bulletin #72. Washington, D.C. Government Printing Office (710 North Capital Street, Washington, D.C. 20407), 1968.

Walker, N. W. *Diet and Salad Suggestions.* Phoenix, Ariz.: Norwalk Press. (P.O. Box 13206, Phoenix, Arizona 85002).

_____ *Raw Vegetable Juices.* New York: Jove Publications, 1977.

Watson, George. *Nutrition and Your Mind.* New York: Harper & Row, 1972.

Watt, Bernice K., Annabel L. Merrill et al. *Composition of Foods: Raw, Processed, Prepared.* U.S.D.A. Handbook #8, 1963. Washington, D.C.: Government Printing Office.

Wigmore, Ann. *Be Your Own Doctor.* Washington, D.C.: Hemisphere Pub.

_____ *Make Your Own Juicer Your Drugstore.* Washington, D.C.: Hemisphere Pub.

Woods, Ralph L. *Government Guides to Health and Nutrition.* New York: Pyramid Books, 1975.

Wordsworth, Jill. *Diet Revolution: Nutrition, Diets and Food Fads— What the Experts Haven't Told You.* New York: St. Martin's Press, 1977.

Yudkin, John. *Sweet and Dangerous.* New York: Bantam Books, 1973.


Beadle, B. W. *Journal of Biological Chemistry,* 149:339.

Beard, F. T. et al. "Effects of Aging and Cooking on the Distribution of Certain Amino Acids and Nitrogen in Beef Muscle." *American Meat Institute Foundation,* 1953, 83:410.

Cheldelin, V. H. et al. *Journal of Nutrition,* 26:477.

Elvehjem, C. A., and Pavcek, P. L. *Modern Hospital,* 61:110.

Farrer, K. T. H. *Australian Chemistry Institute Journal,* "Proceedings" 8:113.

Fritz, J. C. *Poultry Science,* 21:361.

Harris, R. S. *Journal of Nutrition,* 40:367.

_____ *Vitamins & Hormones,* 20:603.

Heller, C. A. et al. *Journal of Nutrition,* 36:377.

Ingelfinger, F. J. "For Want of an Enzyme," *Nutrition Today,* Sept. 1968.

Pottenger, F. M., Jr. "The Effect of Heated Processed Foods and Metabolized Vitamin D Milk on the Dento-Facial Structure of Experimental Animals," *American Journal of Orthodontics and Oral Surgery.*

U.S. Dept. of Agriculture, Human Nutrition Research Branch. *Information Bulletin 112.*

# Index